Biological Rhythms, Sleep and Hypnosis

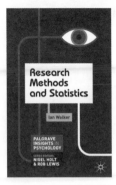
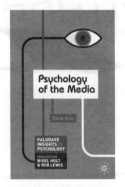
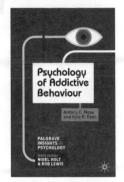
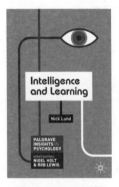
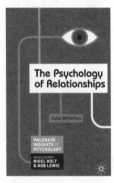
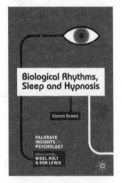
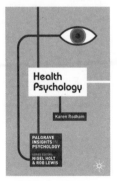
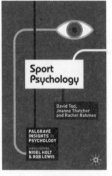
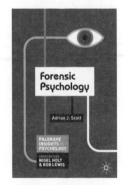
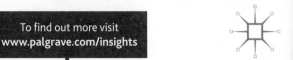

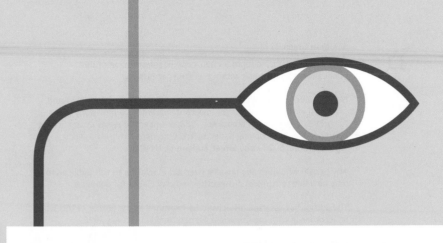

Biological Rhythms, Sleep and Hypnosis

Simon Green

PALGRAVE INSIGHTS IN PSYCHOLOGY

SERIES EDITORS:
NIGEL HOLT & ROB LEWIS

palgrave
macmillan

First published 2011 by
PALGRAVE MACMILLAN

Palgrave Macmillan in the UK is an imprint of Macmillan Publishers Limited,
registered in England, company number 785998, of Houndmills, Basingstoke,
Hampshire RG21 6XS.

Palgrave Macmillan in the US is a division of St Martin's Press LLC,
175 Fifth Avenue, New York, NY 10010.

Palgrave Macmillan is the global academic imprint of the above companies
and has companies and representatives throughout the world.

Palgrave® and Macmillan® are registered trademarks in the United States,
the United Kingdom, Europe and other countries.

ISBN: 978–0–230–25265–3

This book is printed on paper suitable for recycling and made from fully
managed and sustained forest sources. Logging, pulping and manufacturing
processes are expected to conform to the environmental regulations of the
country of origin.

A catalogue record for this book is available from the British Library.

A catalog record for this book is available from the Library of Congress.

10 9 8 7 6 5 4 3 2 1
20 19 18 17 16 15 14 13 12 11

Printed in China

Contents

List of figures and tables

Figures

Table

Note from series editors

Biological rhythms, sleep and hypnosis may collectively be described as part of the study of levels of consciousness, a topic central to the study of psychology. The word consciousness brings to mind words like awareness, understanding and insight. It is clear that this topic is crucial in our study of the science of mind and behaviour.

In this book, Simon Green develops his interest in psychobiology and biological rhythms and includes hypnosis, a subtopic of interest to many. When developing the series of books of which this is part, we looked for topics that needed developing, and we also looked for authors who could not only do the topic justice, but who could adapt their voice to the unique demands of the collection. Green teaches undergraduates and postgraduates while maintaining his knowledge of, and contributing to research in, the area. In addition to this, he is an experienced examiner at principal and chief levels at a major examining board and so has a unique insight into the demands of students and teachers preparing for A-level examinations. His style is direct and knowledgeable, while remaining light and accessible – a great skill, and many of us would like to know how he achieves it.

- *You may be reading this book as part of your preparation for university study.* Simon lectures university students in London. He is aware of the pressures placed on students to keep up with their reading and preparation and has developed a text that provides just the right level of information for developing your skills before entering university.

- *Those reading the book while at university* may be doing so as part of a psychology degree or perhaps as a module within another degree such as nursing or medicine. The range of material here is chosen by us to develop the skills needed at introductory level and Simon's book will undoubtedly inform and interest you.

- *If you are reading the book as part of a pre-university course such as A-level* you will be aware of the material required, perhaps from your chosen textbook or your examination board's detailed psychology specification. Simon has spent time identifying the material required, and has presented it here to help you achieve excellence, either in your learning or teaching. The Reading Guide at the end of the book tells you where different A-level specifications appear.

The subject matter and range covered so eloquently here is such that it will interest readers from a number of disciplines, not just psychology. The material is relevant to biology and physiology to name but two other subjects. Whatever your reason for reading the book, we are sure you will find it interesting, and a useful addition to your library.

NIGEL HOLT AND ROB LEWIS
Series Editors

Chapter 1

Self-awareness, consciousness and biological rhythms

◉ Introduction

In *A Dictionary of Psychology* (Colman, 2001), consciousness is defined as:

> the normal mental condition of the waking state of humans, characterized by the experience of perceptions, thoughts, feelings, awareness of the external world, and often in humans, self-awareness.

In a much earlier, classic text, William James (1890) introduced his now famous phrase 'the stream of consciousness' to refer to the apparently endless flow of such perceptions, thoughts, feelings and images. Basic to our approach to consciousness is the idea of self-awareness; we are 'conscious' of our internal life, and we can report on our thoughts and feelings to others. So self-awareness and consciousness are closely related, but they are not the same thing.

Topics covered in later chapters have a direct or indirect relationship with consciousness and awareness, so we need to outline some psychological approaches to the problems of studying these states.

In this chapter, we will cover:
- Consciousness: general issues
- Conscious and unconscious information processing
- Case studies: consciousness and self-awareness
- Consciousness and awareness
- Consciousness and evolution
- Awareness

⊙ Consciousness: general issues

One simple way to see the difference between consciousness and self-awareness is to look at your, or someone else's, cat or dog. Is the cat conscious? Is it self-aware? Is it aware? We would not normally refer to cats as self-aware, but equally we would not refer to them as 'unconscious'; however, we would happily refer to them as conscious or 'aware', that is, they are clearly responsive to their environment and show alertness and appropriate responses. In fact, with animals, we can reasonably work with just a few terms to describe their states of awareness; awake and alert and fully aware, sleepy and less aware, asleep and unresponsive.

With humans the situation is far more complicated. Whole books (for example Dennett, 1991; Chalmers, 1996; Blackmore, 2003) have been written on the problem of consciousness in humans, and how it can be explained by philosophers and psychologists. In fact, there is no agreed model of consciousness, with major disagreements on whether it can even be studied scientifically at all. To take one example, a central problem in this area is **qualia**. Qualia are our private subjective experience of a particular sensation, for example the smell of coffee, the scent of a rose, the sympathy we feel at the sight of famine sufferers on TV. We can describe these feelings, and others might say they feel the same, but there is no way of knowing whether their experience is exactly the same as ours. Similarly, we cannot 'know' what it is like to be someone else, and in fact we cannot imagine what it would be like to be a cat or a zebra. We cannot know the minds of others.

In theory, we can record the patterns of electrical signals in the brain that represent the coding of an event, the smell of coffee or the smell of roses. But we have no idea how the subjective experience emerges from the brain activity. This is the 'hard problem' of consciousness, 'how physical processes in the brain give rise to subjective experience' (Chalmers, 1995).

Luckily, the major questions of consciousness are not the subject of this book. However, many of the topics do bear indirectly on some of the above issues. Consider, for a moment, the issue of dreams (Chapter 5). Are you conscious and aware in your dreams? In terms of being aware of sensations and perceptions and performing planned actions and behaviours, the answer would be 'yes'. You can also relate the dream content to others (if you remember it), but, crucially, you are also aware that it was a dream and different from waking existence. Apart from the unusual category of lucid dreams (see Chapter 5), we do not have subjective self-awareness in dreams in the sense of being aware it is a dream *during* the dream.

Similarly with hypnosis (Chapter 6). One approach to hypnosis sees it as an 'altered state of consciousness'. Receptive participants under hypnosis seem aware of the world around them, that is, they are conscious. However, their actions may be apparently controlled by the hypnotist, they can, for example, be persuaded to ignore painful stimuli, and have no subjective self-awareness. When brought out of the hypnotized state, they have no recall of their feelings and actions under hypnosis.

Non-dreaming sleep is a different problem. We would accept that we are not conscious during this phase of sleep, and in fact it is the closest, unless we are very unlucky, to unconsciousness that we can get. However, the relationship between dreaming and non-dreaming sleep is intricate and complex (see Chapter 3), and studying them together has led to theories of each.

Do dreams and hypnotic phenomena, when we seem to be conscious but lack self-awareness, represent truly different states of consciousness? One approach that avoids the philosophical complexity of arguments about the nature and definition of consciousness is to look at the patterns of brain activity that underlie these states. The comparison of brain states associated with this is a key element of this text.

◉ Conscious and unconscious information processing

We are much happier talking in terms of our 'self-awareness' than we are of our 'consciousness'. Self-awareness refers to our sense of being in conscious self-control of our behaviour. We can choose to take the bus rather than the train, to have pizza rather than kebabs, to try for a career in finance rather than veterinary science, to move to Australia for better job opportunities. We are also aware of our private thoughts and feelings. In general, we like to think that our daily lives, and in particular our actions and decisions, are under our conscious self-control. In addition, we are uneasy with the sense that our behaviour might be significantly influenced by *unconscious* influences outside our self-awareness.

In fact, it is quite easy to demonstrate that more is going on in our brains than is available to our conscious self-awareness. Think of your first day at infant school. Try to remember what happened, where the classrooms were, who your reception class teacher was, how you felt and

The fact that contemporary views of consciousness link it to controlled processing and focal attention, both of which have limited capacity, is in line with Freud's original view that our conscious life is the tip of the iceberg, with much going on under the surface and outside conscious awareness. In fact, it has been argued that most of our cognitive processing is inaccessible to conscious self-awareness. This in turn raises the interesting question of whether we can be influenced by meaningful stimuli that are not consciously perceived.

Priming and masking

Priming is a popular technique used in experimental cognitive psychology. Two stimuli are presented, one immediately following the other. Responses to the second stimulus, the target, can be influenced by the nature of the first stimulus, the prime. This is especially the case if the two stimuli are words and they are semantically related, that is, having similar meanings or from the same category. For instance, a prime such as 'hospital' speeds up the recognition of a target word such as 'doctor' compared to a target such as 'orange'.

A particular variation of the technique is used to investigate conscious and non-conscious processing – **masking**. If a prime is presented on a computer screen for a very brief time (say 50 msec) and is immediately followed by a mask, such as a meaningless pattern, the participant is not consciously aware of it. However, such masked primes can still influence responses to the target word. Recognition times of semantically related targets are still faster than to unrelated targets. So there is semantic processing (processing for meaning) of the masked prime, that is, processing without awareness.

More impressively, studies have shown that **evoked potential** responses in the brain to the target word vary depending on whether they are semantically related to the masked target, confirming that the primes are being processed in the absence of conscious perception (Kiefer and Brendel, 2006). Reviews of scanning studies involving conscious and unconscious processing of visual stimuli have shown that processing without awareness activates brain regions known to be associated with visual processing, but not areas beyond these regions. Conscious processing activates these same regions, but also leads to increased activity in areas such as the superior parietal and prefrontal cortex (Rees, 2007). This leads to the obvious suggestion that conscious awareness is associated with activity in these regions.

Planning without awareness?

A very different approach has shown equally fascinating findings relating to conscious awareness. We feel that we are in conscious control of our decisions, ranging from deciding to stand up to trying to run the London marathon. However, some studies have cast doubts on this basic assumption. Libet et al. (1983) asked participants to bend their wrists and fingers, and to tell the experimenter whenever they decided to do this. The researchers recorded this time, and also recorded the 'readiness potential' in the **electroencephalograph** (EEG). This is an evoked potential that reliably indexes preparation for movement. They found that the readiness potential *preceded* the *conscious* intention by about 350 msec, and in turn the intention to move preceded the actual movement by about 200 msec.

The bizarre conclusion to this readiness study is that preparation for movement happens *before* we become consciously aware of the intention to move, that is, the brain seems to decide what to do without our conscious control. Libet et al.'s (1983) study can be criticized. It is hard to consistently time participants' conscious decisions to act (note that the key time difference is only about one-third of a second), and the precise relationship between intentions and the readiness potential is not clear. However, a more recent study supports Libet et al.'s conclusions.

Soon et al. (2008) recorded brain activity using **functional magnetic resonance imaging** (fMRI, a popular brain scanning technique), focusing on frontal and parietal cortex. They asked participants to move either their left or right index finger as and when they liked, but to tell the experimenters when they made a decision. The experimenters found that they could predict which finger the participant would move from the specific pattern of activation in frontal and parietal cortex; this was not a huge surprise, as different movements would lead to different patterns of activation. What was astonishing was the finding that they could predict which finger would move by activation patterns occurring *seven* seconds before the participant reported a decision to move the finger, that is, seven seconds before the conscious decision was made. Soon et al. concluded that decisions seem to be sorted out by brain activity some time before we become consciously aware of them; the brain, and not consciousness, is doing all the work.

Psychology, science and society

Soon et al.'s study can be criticized. The decisions are trivial ones, and predictions were not 100% accurate even for these. However, the implications are profound. Responsibility for our actions, whether legal or illegal, relies on our conscious awareness of what we are doing and its implications. If, in fact, it is our brain that is making decisions, with conscious awareness almost an afterthought, how then can people be responsible for their actions?

This particular debate is an aspect of the 'free will/determinism' controversy. Most approaches in psychology are trying to explain how behaviour comes about, that is, how our behaviour is determined, whether it be by biological/genetic, behavioural, social or psychodynamic processes. This aim itself reduces the scope for free will. For instance, when young children commit horrific crimes, we try to explain their behaviour in terms of genetics, early experience, violent video games and so on. It is hard to see such behaviour as the result of free will. However, if psychology eventually eliminates free will, then how do we hold people accountable for their actions? Neuroscientific research such as that by Soon et al. (2008) is adding to the view that we may be far less responsible for our actions than we would like, and in fact even decisions we think are ours are emerging from the unconscious brain. This will become an increasingly important ethical dilemma for society over the coming decades.

◉ Case studies: consciousness and self-awareness

The vegetative state: aware or unaware?

Persistent vegetative state (PVS) can be a consequence of traumatic brain damage, infection, or toxic conditions such as carbon monoxide poisoning. Patients can appear awake, but are unresponsive to any external stimuli and show no apparent awareness of the world around them. They are not conscious, and pose severe ethical dilemmas as they can only be kept alive by 24-hour care, including food and drink, with no clinical hope for recovery. With demand for organ transplants continually increasing, patients' families are often put under pressure to remove life support systems from such patients (Verheijde et al., 2009). The position altered slightly when reports appeared of the occasional patient recovering 'consciousness' after years in PVS. Also, controlled scientific studies have provided additional evidence that more may be going on in PVS than was thought.

Owen et al. (2006) studied a young woman in PVS after a road accident. They asked her (obviously with no behavioural response) to imagine either playing tennis or walking around her house. Using fMRI, they were able to show that these two instructions were associated with different patterns of brain activity. More importantly, tennis was associated with activity in motor areas, and walking around the house with activity in the parahippocampal gyrus (an area of the brain that plays an important role in memory encoding and retrieval); these same areas were activated in control participants asked to imagine the same two activities.

Further studies showed that it was imagining the activity that was crucial, as simply presenting the word 'tennis' did not lead to the same pattern of activation. The authors concluded that this patient was exhibiting conscious awareness and controlled processing of instructions, despite her PVS (Owen and Coleman, 2008). Such processing is highly complex and is unlikely to reflect unconscious processing, but this possibility cannot be excluded, given what we have seen of the brain's capacity for unconscious processing.

The same technique was employed in a recent study involving a large number of patients in either PVS or a 'minimally conscious state' (Monti and Owen, 2010). Five out of 54 patients showed the same pattern of specific brain activation to commands either to imagine being on a tennis court and playing a game of tennis, or to imagine walking from room to room in their house, visualizing anything they could see. The researchers also tried an imaginative extension to the study; patients were asked to answer simple 'yes/no' questions about their family and life by imagining either playing tennis for 'yes' or walking around their house for 'no'. Using the specific patterns of brain activity associated with these measures, the researchers were able to identify 'yes' and 'no' answers to the questions. One patient out of the 54 was able to provide 100% correct answers to questions asked, indicating a high level of cognitive processing and awareness. This patient had been diagnosed as being in PVS.

If a small number of patients in PVS can demonstrate some brain signs of conscious awareness even in the absence of behavioural external signs, the implications are profound. It raises the possibility that other patients in PVS have similar states of awareness and to treat them as effectively the 'living dead' is ethically and legally wrong. Of course, it does seem that only a tiny fraction of such patients will show such awareness, and we cannot know whether this is associated with conscious self-awareness, although many researchers in the area believe that it does. Others are sceptical of the use of measures of brain activity to assess 'consciousness' and feel that wider ethical issues are involved (Kitzinger and Kitzinger, 2010).

The split brain and conscious awareness

Epilepsy is a result of a violent and uncontrolled electrical discharge in the brain. The source may be a developing tumour or cyst, or scar tissue following brain surgery. In these cases, the epilepsy is said to have a 'focus'. In other cases, the condition has no apparent focus. Where a focus can be identified, it may be possible to remove it surgically. In other cases, epileptic attacks can be controlled using anticonvulsant drugs. In rare cases, the epilepsy is disabling – full blown epilepsy ('grand mal') leads to temporary unconsciousness – with several attacks each day, and is unresponsive to drugs.

If a focus cannot be identified in such cases, an alternative operation is possible. Devised in the 1940s, this involved cutting the major pathway, the **corpus callosum**, between the two cerebral hemispheres. Doing this confined the epileptic discharge to one hemisphere, thus preventing its spread to the opposite hemisphere, and so reducing the severity of attacks. The technical term for the operation is a **commissurotomy** but it has gone down in history as the 'split brain' operation, although, technically, the brain is not split into two hemispheres; they are still connected low down in the brainstem and, in most **split brain patients**, small pathways still connect the hemispheres.

In the first studies, the operation seemed to have a clear clinical benefit in reducing the severity of the epilepsy, with no apparent side effects. This was a surprise as the operation cuts the major pathway connecting the two hemispheres. In fact, the facetious suggestion was made that the only function of the corpus callosum was to hold the two hemispheres together. However, in the 1950s, Roger Sperry, one of the legendary figures of psychology, began his investigations into the split brain and its effects (he won the Nobel prize in 1981). Sperry devised a method of presenting visual stimuli to only one hemisphere at a time.

Using the anatomy of the pathways, he realized that a stimulus presented out to the right of a participant looking straight ahead (the right visual field, RVF) was transmitted directly to the left hemisphere, while a stimulus presented out to the left of the participant (left visual field, LVF) went directly to the right hemisphere. In normal people, the information then passes rapidly through the corpus callosum to the opposite hemisphere, but in the split brain patient, it was confined to the target hemisphere.

Using his **divided field technique** and working with split brain patients, Sperry was able to show that words presented in the RVF were rapidly perceived and read out, while those presented in the LVF went unreported and unrecognized. Why was this? Words presented in the RVF go to the left hemisphere. In most people, this contains the language system, so these words can be identified and read out. (The more specialized functions of the two hemispheres are that the left hemisphere processes language, maths and logic, while the right hemisphere processes visuospatial abilities, face recognition, visual imagery and music.) Words presented in the LVF go to the right hemisphere. With no language system, this cannot read or report the word presented, and in these patients, the words cannot pass to the left hemisphere. In fact, the split brain patient shows no awareness of the words at all.

A simpler way of demonstrating this *dissociation* is to blindfold the patient and give them objects to hold in each hand. Nerve pathways from each hand project to the opposite hemisphere. The normal participant can tell you if they are the same and what each one is, for example an apple and a banana, as the hemispheres cooperate through the corpus callosum. The split brain patient can tell you what they are holding in the right hand, as this goes to the left hemisphere and its language system. They cannot tell you what they are holding in the left hand, which goes to the right hemisphere, or whether it is the same as the object in the right hand, and in fact will show no awareness that they are holding anything in the left hand at all.

The right hemisphere does have one response outlet; it controls the left hand. Sperry was able to show that the right hemisphere could read simple nouns, and use the left hand to select the appropriate object from a selection. It was also superior to the right hemisphere at processing faces and other visuospatial stimuli – given a choice of faces, the participant would select the one presented to the right hemisphere rather than the one presented to the left hemisphere. However, crucially, the split brain patient could not comment on or explain what was going on when his left hand selected an object; in fact they would sometimes deny that it was their hand doing the actions.

Studies with split brain patients by Sperry (1964) and Gazzaniga (Sperry and Gazzaniga,1967) have emphasized how human consciousness and self-awareness are dependent on language. When we ask participants to report what they see, or how they feel, they have to use the left hemisphere language system. Similarly, when we talk to others about our feelings and ambitions, or reflect quietly on how life is going, or simply think, we use our left hemisphere language system. We also have access to what is going on in the right hemisphere via the corpus callosum, so we feel fully integrated as a single personality. The split brain patient experiences life very differently. When asked about their thoughts and feelings, they are reporting from their left hemisphere, as the right hemisphere has no verbal outlet for any thoughts or feelings it may have, or for the high-level visuospatial processing it can do. It can impose itself in some ways; one split brain patient reported that she would choose one set of clothes with her right hand (left hemisphere), while her left hand (right hemisphere) would choose an entirely different set.

More bizarrely, one split brain patient turned out to have reasonable language abilities in both hemispheres. Using a variation of the divided field, researchers were able to ask each hemisphere various questions (the right hemisphere answered by arranging scrabble letters with the left hand) and found some intriguing differences; for instance, the left hemisphere's ambition was to be a draughtsman, while the right hemisphere wanted to be a racing driver.

From split brain research, Sperry concluded that the two hemispheres in fact reflect different types of consciousness, although this is probably going far beyond the data. Only about a dozen split brain patients have been intensively tested, and all have had severe epileptic conditions for years before long-term drug therapy and major brain surgery. Generalizing to the normal population would not be justified.

The split brain studies do, however, demonstrate some important features of awareness. They show that our conscious self-awareness is almost completely dependent on language. In the intact person, the left hemisphere language system can comment on all brain activities, in both left and right hemispheres, as they are connected via the corpus callosum. The split brain patient can only comment on the activities of the left hemisphere, as the right hemisphere is disconnected from the language system. Yet the right hemisphere continues to process information, supporting the conclusion from priming and readiness studies reviewed earlier that a great deal of processing in the brain can take place out of conscious awareness.

Blindsight

The visual pathways from the retina in the eye to the brain run to the primary visual cortex in the occipital lobe at the back of the brain. There is a primary visual area at the back of each hemisphere, and the arrangement of the visual pathways, outlined previously in relation to Sperry's split brain studies, is highly systematic. With eyes focused straight ahead, the area to our right, or the right visual field, projects to the left hemisphere, and the left visual field projects to the right hemisphere.

Because of this arrangement, the effects of brain damage to the visual cortex are predictable. Loss of the visual cortex in one hemisphere leads to loss of vision in one half of the visual field (called homonymous hemianopia). Although examples are rare, one patient in particular has provided fascinating insights into cognitive processing without awareness. Known by his initials, DB, he had a tumour growing in his right visual cortex, and the only treatment was to surgically remove the visual cortex. This left DB effectively 'blind' in his left visual field (hemifield).

In the 1970s, Weiskrantz began a series of studies with DB to test whether he had any residual vision in his 'blind' hemifield (Weiskrantz et al., 1974; Weiskrantz, 2002). It turned out that when presented with visual stimuli in his left hemifield, DB showed better than chance performance in saying whether something had been presented. Even more impressively, he could point at where the stimulus was, or whether it was moving or not. Studies with other patients show that they can identify facial expressions at above chance levels. Note the key element of these studies – the patient is subjectively blind, and is effectively *guessing* when asked to identify objects in the blind hemifield.

This phenomenon is known as **blindsight**, and is another example of high-level cognitive processing without awareness. We know that there are pathways from the retina of each eye to higher visual centres that bypass the primary visual cortex, and these are probably responsible for the residual unconscious visual processing in the blind hemifield.

👁 Consciousness and awareness

The evidence from studies with normal participants and patients with brain damage reinforce the view that complex cognitive processing can occur in the absence of conscious awareness. Can this help us devise a simple system for categorizing states of awareness?

Edelman (1992) proposes a simple but popular view:

- **Primary consciousness** refers to straightforward awareness of the world, of sensations and perceptions. There is no 'self-awareness'. This is how we might describe animal awareness, or the dreaming and hypnotic states in humans.
- **Higher order consciousness** refers to subjective self-awareness, the sense of knowing we are conscious, that our thoughts and actions are ours; we are conscious of being conscious. This gives us a sense of self, of past and future, and is based on the development of the self-concept. This is what distinguishes humans from other animals, although recent work on self-awareness and theory of mind in great apes means that this distinction may not be as absolute as was once thought.

Another term for subjective self-awareness is **metarepresentation**. The brains of all animals form a representation of the world they inhabit; if they didn't, they could not operate effectively in that world. Metarepresentation is one step up; it is our ability to represent ourselves as we operate in the world, to reflect on our actions and decisions, and to know that we are an individual among a world of individuals.

Of course, a simple categorization leaves open all the philosophical questions about the nature of conscious self-awareness, and, in particular, how it emerges from brain function. Another question is, what is conscious self-awareness for?

👁 Consciousness and evolution

Psychology has happily taken on board the neo-Darwinian view that we are the products of biological evolution, particularly from the time that humans branched off from other primates about 6 million years ago. A basic assumption is that specifically human characteristics, including conscious self-awareness, must give us an evolutionary advantage over other animals.

There are, of course, many speculations. Humphrey (1986), for example, feels that it is tied in with our social lives. Self-awareness means that we know what it is like to be human, but more than that, it enables us to make intelligent guesses about other people; this is the area of psychology known as **social cognition**. By being self-aware, that is, by thinking about our own thoughts and feelings, and by assuming others are doing the same, we can apply our self-knowledge or 'theory of mind' to understand and predict the behaviour of others. This then allows for complex social interaction and the development of modern human societies. There are also convincing arguments that some disorders, such as autism and schizophrenia, may involve a failure in self-awareness and metarepresentation, leading to problems with social communication.

There are other ideas. Self-awareness allows us to consider courses of action, to plan for the future in the light of past experience. Animals with only primary consciousness have a limited and probably hard-wired capacity to consider future events and to foresee the consequences of their actions. This ability to plan ahead would be a crucial advantage for humans over the rest of the animal world. However, we have also seen that much of our cognitive processing, even decision making, takes place outside conscious awareness, so it seems that our self-awareness is, in fact, of limited capacity.

Ideas on the functions of consciousness are only speculations. They depend on 'consciousness' being selected through the same evolutionary processes as our other specifically human characteristics, such as walking upright or sophisticated language. But this assumption leads in turn back to the nature of conscious self-awareness. How is it wired into the brain? We saw earlier that by comparing conscious with unconscious processing of stimuli, we can identify areas, such as prefrontal cortex, that seem to be activated during the conscious aware state. It may be that consciousness emerges and is selected for when a brain becomes sufficiently complex in terms of numbers of cells and organization. This leads to the interesting speculation that a sufficiently complex artificial brain, that is, a robot, could achieve conscious self-awareness.

But even if we identify brain areas and organization crucial to consciousness, we still have no idea how the subjective experiences (qualia) emerge from the 'wet stuff' of brain matter – neurons and their interconnections. This is the truly philosophical aspect of consciousness; the words we use to talk about it have no immediate relationship with the technical terms we use to describe brain structure and function, because the brain is physical and consciousness is not physical.

So we are left with many unanswered questions about this fascinating topic, although many brilliant psychologists and philosophers have tried to answer them. The outline presented in this chapter serves as a background to much of the material in this book, as sleep states, dreams and hypnosis all involve variations in states of primary and higher order consciousness. However, humans, along with all living things, are also biological organisms and subject to rhythmic changes in arousal and alertness. To understand sleep as an altered state of awareness, we need to put it into the context of biological rhythms. However, before we can do this we need to look at how we can measure states of awareness and what this tells us about the brain mechanisms involved.

◉ Awareness

We have already discussed the key concept of 'awareness' or primary consciousness. 'Awareness' refers to the capacity to respond to outside events, that is, to register them and to show an appropriate response. The fully awake human is fully aware, while we would consider the deeply asleep human to be unaware or unconscious. Awareness is closely associated with the state of the brain, and we shall see that electrical patterns in the brain can be used to index different states of awareness (Chapter 3).

This brings us to hypnosis, which has been a controversial area. The idea that people can be put into a particular suggestible state and then be made to follow the hypnotist's instructions is appealing to some, and ridiculous to others. In fact, hypnosis is not confined to stage shows; it is used in some therapeutic settings to help clients recall so-called 'repressed memories' from the distant past. In theory, this allows the client to understand their early experiences, which in turn may help to resolve current psychological difficulties.

The link to awareness, sleep and biological rhythms is that one major theory of hypnosis sees it as a 'different state of awareness', in the same way that deep sleep is seen as a specific and measurable state of awareness. An alternative approach does not see hypnosis as a special state, but instead tries to explain hypnotic phenomena using established psychological principles. We know that other states of awareness, such as waking and sleeping, can be distinguished through different patterns of brain electrical activity. So a key test of the 'hypnosis as a distinct state of awareness' hypothesis would be to show that the hypnotic state is associated with a distinctive pattern of brain activity. This is explored in Chapter 6.

Measuring states of awareness

Most measures of different states of awareness depend upon the electrical activity of the brain. The brain is made up of cells called **neurons**. Neurons are elongated cells that are specialized to transmit small electrical impulses along their length. These impulses, known as **nerve impulses** or action potentials, represent information transmission in the brain. It is a surprising fact that everything the brain does is represented, or coded, as patterns of these nerve impulses. When we see, hear, smell or taste, all these sensations are coded as electrical activity in particular parts of the brain. Similarly, our cognitive abilities such as attention, perception, learning and memory all depend upon nerve impulses being transmitted along neurons.

We can record the brain's electrical activity using special recording electrodes. In research with animals, we can actually insert tiny electrodes into different parts of the brain and record their activity. For instance, if animals are shown different objects, then electrodes in the visual parts of the brain record an increase in electrical activity. If they hear sounds, then activity increases in the parts of the brain dealing with sound (auditory cortex). Incidentally, as we know the brain operates using an electrical code, we can also stimulate activity artificially using electrodes. In some cases, this is done in humans as part of a checking process before brain surgery, to make sure the operation will not damage essential structures. Human patients report visual and auditory sensations if stimulated in visual or auditory parts of the brain, as well as more complex experiences such as emotional feelings if stimulation is in deeper brain areas.

The most common types of electrical recording in humans do not involve inserting electrodes into the brain. Instead, electrodes are placed on the surface of the head (this is called a 'non-invasive' procedure; inserting electrodes into the brain would be an 'invasive' procedure). A network of electrodes (usually between 24 and 64) is used to record activity from many parts of the brain simultaneously. As the brain is made up of somewhere between 10 and 100 billion neurons, this procedure records electrical activity from many millions of neurons simultaneously. Because of this, the initial pattern looks highly complex and meaningless. However, nowadays, the data is fed into a computer, and this can identify patterns in the recordings over time.

This recording technique is known as the electroencephalograph (EEG). Since its introduction in the 1930s, it has been crucial to our understanding of brain function, and in particular to the study of states of awareness.

EEG patterns: synchronized and desynchronized

Electrical activity, as recorded by the EEG, has two key characteristics that can be measured. *Amplitude* represents the amount or intensity of electrical activity, while *frequency* refers to the speed of activity. In addition, EEG recordings can be divided into two basic forms:

- In a **synchronized EEG**, we can identify regular wave patterns. As we shall see with the stages of sleep, a regular wave pattern will have a characteristic amplitude and, especially, frequency. Alpha waves, for instance, are seen in the drowsy brain; they are relatively low amplitude and have a frequency of between 8 and 12 waves (or cycles) per second. This latter measure – cycles per second – is also known as 'herz'.

  As any EEG recording represents the activity of many millions of neurons, a synchronized pattern must mean that the majority of these neurons are working *in phase*. We know that the brain is made up of many different structures and pathways that have different roles in the brain's many activities. Therefore we would not expect them to operate in phase except under special circumstances; these include the stages of sleep and some forms of drug or damage-induced coma.

- In a **desynchronized EEG**, there is no identifiable and regular wave pattern. During waking activity, the brain's many structures and pathways are actively processing a vast amount and variety of information. We would not expect them to be working in phase, and indeed they are not. Overall, the EEG also has low amplitude and high frequency.

So we can describe two basic types of EEG. The synchronized EEG, typically found in some stages of sleep, has an identifiable wave form that can be defined by a characteristic amplitude and frequency. The desynchronized EEG does not have an identifiable wave form, but can be defined in terms of its general amplitude and frequency. The alert waking brain is characterized by a fast desynchronized EEG.

Research into human sleep has relied heavily on the EEG. It has also been used in the study of hypnosis. As we shall see, one approach to hypnosis tries to identify changes in the EEG that correspond with the hypnotic state (Chapter 6). If these were found, it would support the theory that hypnosis is a special state of brain arousal or awareness.

The EEG and behaviour

The EEG provides an excellent index of general brain arousal. If we were shown EEG records, we would immediately identify a fast desynchronized pattern as being associated with an aroused brain and alert waking behaviour. If the EEG record was dominated by slow waves of high amplitude, we would conclude that this was from a sleeping brain. There can be significant exceptions to this relationship between the EEG and behaviour. REM sleep (Chapter 3), one of the stages of sleep, is associated with a fast desynchronized EEG although the person is deeply asleep, that is, the brain is highly active, but this is not shown in observable behaviour. So while the EEG is always a reliable index of brain activation, we do have to be cautious in assuming it also reflects behavioural activation.

We should also note that the same non-invasive recording technique can be used to study information processing in the brain. If specific stimuli are repeatedly presented, they elicit an evoked potential in the EEG. Computer averaging of the responses reveals the evoked potential as a characteristic waveform that stands out from the background EEG pattern. Evoked potentials have been extensively used in the study of attention and in investigating the brain mechanisms underlying the processing of, for example, words and emotional face expressions.

Mechanisms of brain arousal

We know that the EEG is generated by the activity of the brain's neurons. An aroused EEG reflects the high arousal of millions of neurons, while the synchronized EEG is produced by the relatively low arousal of neurons working in phase together. What contributes to the arousal state of the brain?

Although neurons are active all the time, they are particularly so when processing information. When we are awake, we are taking in information from our visual, auditory and other senses. The areas of the brain dealing with learning and memory, language, planning and emotions will use this sensory input in their own processing. The brain will be aroused and the EEG desynchronized.

It was initially assumed that it was the sensory input that kept the brain aroused (the historical work on brain mechanisms of arousal is reviewed in Wickens, 2009). During waking behaviour, this input is maintained at a high level and leads to correspondingly high levels of brain activity. At night, sensory input falls, brain arousal falls, and a state of sleep follows. This was the passive theory of sleep, that it is a natural state of the brain when sensory input falls below a certain level.

However, in a series of dramatic studies in the 1950s and 60s by researchers such as Moruzzi and Magoun (1965), this theory was shown to be wrong. It was known that a key role in brain arousal was played by a network of millions of neurons buried deep in the brain, known as the reticular formation or **ascending reticular activating system** (ARAS; see Figure 1.1). Stimulation of this structure in cats and rats led to an aroused desynchronized EEG and behavioural activation. Lesions or damage to the ARAS led to a sleep-like state. Although the ARAS received inputs from most of our sensory systems, this still did not mean that sensory input was not the crucial factor in sleeping and waking; importantly, further studies showed that the ARAS still controlled brain arousal even when it was *disconnected* from all sensory input.

Thinking scientifically

These studies might well not be allowed under today's ethical guidelines for animal research. Disconnecting the ARAS from sensory input involved sectioning or cutting through the brain just above the spinal cord. These experiments could not be done on humans, and even in animals there was no possibility of the cat or rat surviving. Even stimulating the ARAS involved implanting electrodes deep into the brain of anaesthetized animals, then allowing them to wake up. To repeat these studies today would require an extremely powerful scientific argument to justify the suffering of the animals involved.

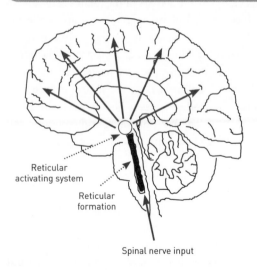

Reticular
activating system

Reticular
formation

Spinal nerve input

Figure 1.1 ARAS and brainstem areas

One of the most important figures in the history of sleep research was Jouvet (1967). He developed the research on the arousal function of the ARAS, with a specific focus on its role in sleep. He was able to show that there are specific centres (known as nuclei) buried within the ARAS that control various aspects of sleep and arousal. We shall meet some of these in Chapter 3, but at this stage there are two important points to make:

1　Stimulation of certain nuclei in the ARAS can produce sleep in awake animals. This means that sleep is not passive, but an active state imposed on the brain by these sleep centres.

2　The discovery of the ARAS and its functions altered our approach to the understanding of relationships between brain arousal and behavioural arousal. Although brain arousal, via the ARAS, is sensitive to sensory input, there can be times when the ARAS and the centres it contains regulate brain arousal patterns independently of sensory input. These will be times when brain arousal measured using the EEG might be decoupled from behavioural activation. An example would be rapid eye movement (REM) sleep, when an aroused EEG pattern is associated with behavioural sleep.

The pioneering research of Dement, Kleitman and Aserinsky into the nature of sleep (see Chapter 3) took place through the 1950s and 60s. The neurophysiological studies outlined above on the functions of the ARAS in sleep and arousal were running in parallel. This meant that by the time we reached the 1970s, the whole picture of sleep and arousal had changed. There were different phases of sleep, controlled by a complex network of brain centres and pathways. The experience of sleep can seem simple – go to bed, fall asleep, wake up – but it is underpinned by a sophisticated balance of arousing and inhibiting influences from a variety of brain areas. Since then, research has built on these findings to provide an even more detailed picture of how the brain interacts with the world outside to control arousal states such as sleep and other biological rhythms. The arousal system of the brain will be involved in all states of consciousness and awareness, such as dreaming and hypnosis.

Summary

- Although introduced into psychology by Freud over 100 years ago, consciousness has only recently become an acceptable topic for scientific study. Before the term became widely used by scientists, consciousness was seen to be equivalent to controlled information processing or focal attention.

- Primary consciousness, or basic awareness, is a property of animals and perhaps the dreaming or hypnotized human. Higher order consciousness or metarepresentation is the complex self-awareness found only in humans.

- We have no idea how self-awareness emerges from brain activity, and this is one of the great philosophical and psychological problems to be solved.

- There is evidence from a variety of experimental psychological studies and from research with brain-damaged patients that self-awareness is not essential for high-level information processing. We are constantly influenced by brain processes that are unconscious and of which we are completely unaware.

- The study of arousal and awareness is fundamental to understanding consciousness. Besides obvious states of awareness such as being asleep and being awake, there are more controversial ones such as dreaming sleep and hypnosis.

- States of awareness can be correlated with the electrical activity of the brain, recorded using the electroencephalograph (EEG).

- The two basic EEG patterns are a fast desynchronized pattern associated with brain arousal and a slow synchronized pattern associated with drowsiness and sleep. Behaviour and the EEG are often correlated, but they can be dissociated, as in REM or dreaming sleep.

- Control of brain arousal involves the ascending reticular activating system (ARAS), which originates in the brainstem. Although this can respond to sensory input, it can increase or decrease brain arousal independently of other factors. Classic studies and more recent research show that sleep is not a purely passive phenomenon, but is an active state imposed on the brain by a complex network of centres and pathways.

Chapter 2

Biological rhythms

👁 Introduction

The natural world is full of rhythms, patterns of activity. The sea has high and low tides each day. Some plants, such as morning glory, flower regularly, but only in the evenings. Some beach-living worms burrow down when the tide comes in, and emerge when it goes out again. The human female menstrual rhythm is a regular monthly cycle. Many animals hibernate each winter. As the cold weather approaches, these animals prepare by laying down extra body fat and becoming less active. Day-living (**diurnal**) animals sleep when it becomes dark and awake when morning arrives. Night-living (**nocturnal**) animals are alert and active at night and sleep during daylight.

Humans are diurnal creatures, accustomed to sleeping at night-time and staying awake during daylight hours. Even during sleep, we can identify rhythmic activity; humans and many other animals show a regular oscillation between different phases of sleep, including periods of 'dreaming' sleep.

We can therefore identify literally thousands of rhythms across the living world. Some, such as the stages of sleep, occur in less than 24 hours; this frequency, or periodicity, is known as **ultradian**. The majority of biological rhythms have a periodicity of 24 hours, and these are known as **circadian**. Rhythms taking longer than 24 hours are known generally as **infradian** rhythms, with those such as hibernation, with a periodicity of one year, known as **circannual**.

This chapter will be describing many of these rhythms, focusing on why they evolved and how they are controlled. We will concentrate on sleep in particular, partly because it has been the most researched, and partly because it is the most fascinating. In humans, sleep has always been a mystery, a period of apparent 'unconsciousness' and non-reactivity, but including phases of dreaming whose meaning has baffled investigators for centuries and whose relationship to consciousness and awareness is still debated.

Apart from the nature of biological rhythms and their control mechanisms, there are a number of other interesting aspects. As living organisms, we have our own set of biological rhythms, the most obvious one being our sleep–waking cycle. However, unlike animals, we do not always let them guide our behaviour, for example trying to work when we should be asleep. What are the consequences of trying to go against these biological drives?

> **In this chapter, we will cover:**
> - Free-running biological rhythms
> - Different types of biological rhythms
> - Endogenous pacemakers
> - Disrupting biological rhythms

We noted above some examples of the wide range of biological rhythms found in the living world. Why should they exist at all?

Plants and animals live in particular environments. Animals may be day or night living – diurnal or nocturnal – while plants occupy a range of habitats across the globe. However, wherever they live, plants and animals are subject to regular changes in their environments. The most obvious one is the alternation of day and night over each 24-hour day. Additionally, there are the different seasons – spring, summer, autumn, winter in temperate zones such as Europe and the USA. Each season is associated with changes in temperature and day length, both of which can affect plants and animals. Beach-living plants and animals are also subject to tides – some algae come to the surface when the tide is out and burrow down when it comes in.

These environmental variations are caused by the fact that the earth rotates through 360^0 once every 24 hours, and, over the course of one year, completes one orbit of the sun. It has been doing this since before living organisms evolved, and it seems that evolution has built mechanisms into plants and animals that allow them to adapt to these changing conditions. We can show this through laboratory studies.

◉ Free-running biological rhythms

It seems obvious that the behaviour of plants and animals can be controlled by rhythmic changes in the outside world. But a central question is whether they are completely at the mercy of the environment, and dependent, for instance, on the change from light to dark in order to trigger sleep. A simple way to test this is to remove possible environmental triggers and see what happens. Such studies are called 'free running', as biological rhythms are observed in the absence of environmental stimuli or cues.

Such studies have a long history. The earliest recorded was in 1729, when French astronomer Jean de Mairan observed that the heliotrope, a plant whose leaves open during the day and close at night, maintained this pattern even when kept in continuous dark. What does this imply? Seen under normal conditions, we might conclude that the heliotrope is sensitive to the effects of light, opening its leaves when morning comes and closing them as darkness falls. But the fact that it maintains this pattern in constant dark means that the heliotrope must have an inbuilt, or **endogenous**, mechanism that regulates leaf opening and closing in the absence of light.

By now, many hundreds of such free-running studies have been done, across the living world, and results are consistent. The beach-living algae mentioned earlier show the same rhythmic pattern, of burrowing into the sand when the tide comes in and emerging as it goes out, even when kept in laboratory conditions with no tides present. The timing of their burrowing and emerging in the laboratory matches the timing of tidal flows at their home beach. Species of squirrel that hibernate show a regular annual (yearly) pattern of storing fat reserves and reducing body temperature during the autumn, in preparation for hibernation over winter. They show this same annual pattern if kept in the laboratory in constant light and temperature conditions.

The internal mechanisms that allow biological rhythms to persist even when the normal environmental stimuli (for example light, temperature) are absent are referred to as **endogenous pacemakers**, **body clocks** or endogenous clocks. They are inbuilt or genetic systems. One interesting early observation was that they are not that accurate. The heliotrope in the laboratory opens and closes its leaves at roughly 22-hour intervals, not 24, and as we shall see, the same applies to the human sleep–waking cycle.

In the normal world, biological rhythms are maintained in synchrony with the outside world of light and dark, tidal flows and so on. Yet the endogenous pacemakers are not perfectly accurate, and if it was up to them, heliotropes would have open leaves at midnight, algae would eventually drown, and we would be fast asleep at midday. So other factors must be involved, and these are the environmental stimuli themselves. Research has shown that stimuli such as light and dark, temperature and so on play a key role in the precise synchronization of biological rhythms with the outside world, so that heliotropes open and close leaves at the right time and we sleep at night and wake in the morning. These environmental stimuli that play a key role in the synchronization of biological rhythms are called **exogenous** (outside) **zeitgebers** (from the German, meaning time-giver), or zeitgebers for short.

Studying scientifically → Siffre's (1975) cave study

So far we have looked at studies in plants and animals. Would similar effects be found in humans, with their vastly more complex brains? In another of those case studies that have had such an influence on psychology, French geologist Michel Siffre volunteered for an experiment in free-running biological rhythms. He spent 179 days in a specially prepared underground cave in Texas. The cave was kept at a steady temperature of 70^0. Siffre could use a telephone to ask for the artificial lights to be switched off when he wanted to sleep, and to be put on when he awoke. Before he slept, Siffre attached himself to recording equipment that monitored his sleep patterns and other physiological measures such as body temperature, heart rate and blood pressure.

Two important findings emerged from this study. First, Siffre's normal 24-hour sleep–waking cycle extended to between 25 and 32 hours, so his days effectively became longer. Although he was in the cave for 179 days, on Siffre's own body clock, it was only the 151st day. This is in line with the free-running studies on plants and animals; in the absence of light as a zeitgeber, the endogenous pacemaker can regulate our circadian rhythm of sleeping and waking, but not precisely in tune with the outside world.

Second, Siffre's body temperature also maintained its circadian rhythm. It extended to about 25 hours, but remained more consistent than the sleep–waking cycle. This meant that eventually body temperature and the sleep–waking cycle, which are usually in phase, became decoupled, a state known as 'internal desynchronization'. We normally fall asleep in the evening as body temperature is falling, and wake in the morning when it is rising. Siffre would have been sleeping at different points of the temperature cycle. This desynchronization also means that we must have at least two independent biological pacemakers or body clocks, one for the sleep–waking cycle and one for body temperature.

Siffre suffered some serious psychological problems during his long period of isolation. By the 80th day, he was reporting feelings of depression and suicidal thoughts, and performing badly on simple tests of memory and manual dexterity (hand skill). These effects could not be attributed to sleep deprivation, as he could sleep as much as he liked. They are more likely to have been caused by the internal desyn-chronization of biological rhythms; as we shall see, the disruption of rhythms associated with shiftwork and jet lag can lead to serious physical and psychological health problems.

Siffre continued to have mild psychological problems for some months after the study ended, but clearly had some fond memories of his time in the cave, as in 1999 he took part in a similar study in the French alps.

Psychology as science

Siffre's cave study has entered psychology's folklore, but it is important not to get too carried away. With only one participant we would need to be very cautious in generalizing the conclusions to the wider population, and if Siffre's was the only study on free-running circadian rhythms, we would consider it suggestive rather than conclusive. However, the key point is that it is only one study among many, so we can look at the overall picture to see if findings are consistent across different studies. This is a critical part of the scientific process. Any single study or experiment can often be criticized, for weak methodology or perhaps because of gender or cultural bias. What is far more important is whether a number of studies in the same area produce results that are consistent.

Siffre's study was a single case study and on its own we could not draw strong conclusions on the roles of body clocks and zeitgebers. However, the findings are entirely in line with previous work on plants and animals. In free-running conditions, circadian rhythms are maintained by the internal body clock, but slightly out of synchrony with the normal 24-hour light–dark cycle, usually lengthening to 25 hours or more. Even more convincingly, other studies on free-running rhythms in human partici-pants have provided similar results. Aschoff (1967) used a more controlled environment, a custom-built laboratory in a basement in Germany, and groups of volunteer participants. He found that, as with Siffre, circadian rhythms of sleep–waking and body temperature became longer than 24 hours, averaging about 25 hours. Again in line with Siffre, body temperature maintained a more consistent rhythm than sleep–waking, which could vary between 22 hours – a shortening of the 'biological' day – and 28 hours – a lengthening of the day.

So, findings across a range of studies are consistent and support the picture of biological rhythms outlined earlier. Our endogenous pacemakers, or body clocks, provide a basic circadian rhythm for a variety of behavioural and physiological processes. However, it is crucial that biological rhythms are synchronized with the light–dark, day–night cycles of the natural world. This is achieved through the action of light as a zeitgeber. The onset of light in the morning and the transition from light to dark in the evening act as triggers for the daily resetting of the endogenous body clocks.

By now, we know a great deal about the mechanisms behind the interaction of pacemakers and zeitgebers, and we deal with this aspect of sleep–waking later. At this stage, it is important to understand the widespread nature of this basic aspect of biological rhythms in living organisms. Biological rhythms are inbuilt, but rely on zeitgebers for precise synchronization with the outside world.

Before looking at research into sleep, the following section outlines the different categories of biological rhythm found in the living world.

⊙ Different types of biological rhythms

Circadian rhythms

Circadian rhythms have a periodicity of 24 hours. The best known is the sleep–waking cycle, with one period of each in 24 hours. However, it has been estimated that there are over 100 physiological systems in the body that exhibit a circadian rhythm. Body temperature has one peak and one trough every 24 hours, being at its lowest in the early morning and its highest in the afternoon. Most hormones in the body show a diurnal pattern, as do the chemicals in the brain known as 'neurotransmitters', which play a vital part in communication between brain cells (neurons).

These examples show the central role of light and dark as zeitgebers. Most animals are diurnal, awake and alert in the day and asleep at night. Some are nocturnal, sleeping during the day but awake and alert at night. Either way, animals have adapted to environmental conditions. For diurnal animals, being awake with an increasing body temperature and hormonal activity during the day allows for increased physiological arousal and energy expenditure. At night, when active behaviour is impossible, sleep is imposed by the endogenous pacemakers and sleep centres, and body temperature falls in line with the body's physiological activity. The reverse pattern operates for nocturnal animals. In each case, light onset in the morning and the arrival of darkness at night act as crucial zeitgebers, synchronizing biological rhythms with the environment.

Infradian rhythms

Infradian rhythms are biological rhythms that have a periodicity of more than one day. The name derives from the Latin for 'less than one day', as there is less than one cycle in 24 hours. Examples include the human female menstrual cycle, with an average length of 28 days (menses, another name for menstruation, derives from the Latin for 'month'), and hibernation in many animals such as squirrels and bears. Hibernation is an example of a biological rhythm with a periodicity of one year – these are also known as circannual ('about one year') rhythms.

Both the menstrual cycle and hibernation involve complex changes in the physiology of the body, which must be controlled by centres in the brain, that is, there must be endogenous pacemakers specifically linked to these infradian rhythms.

Infradian rhythms such as hibernation are clearly designed to help animals adapt to environmental conditions. During winter, it is difficult to find food, so hibernating can be a sensible response, but it also means that hibernation must be in synchrony with the outside world to be effective; there would be no point in hibernating during the autumn and waking up as winter approaches. We have already seen that squirrels kept in constant laboratory conditions still show the appropriate pattern of physiological responses, so hibernation must be controlled by endogenous pacemakers in the brain. However, in the same way that the rhythm of sleeping and waking is perfectly synchronized with the falling of darkness in the evening and the onset of light in the morning, so hibernation is synchronized with the onset of winter by changes in the outside temperature and the short-ening of daylight hours associated with the winter months.

The infradian menstrual cycle is different. It is under the control of hormones released from the pituitary gland, which lies in the cranial (skull) cavity, connected to the hypothalamus at the base of the brain, and under the direct control of this brain structure. The average cycle length is 28 days, although it can vary from 20 to 40 days. In most women, the cycle is quite regular, suggesting that the internal control by endogenous pacemakers is the dominant mechanism, with exogenous zeitgebers playing little or no part.

However, there do seem to be conditions where the menstrual cycle can be modified by external stimuli. It has been a frequent observation throughout history that the menstrual cycles of women, such as nuns, who live for extended periods in closed communities tend to synchronize, that is, tend to occur at the same time. A fascinating study by Russell et al. (1980) identified a role for exogenous zeitgebers in this phenomenon. If sweat from one woman was rubbed onto the upper lip of a second woman, over a period of time their menstrual cycles would synchronize. Russell et al. concluded that **pheromones** played a key role in this synchronization. Pheromones are chemicals found in tiny traces in animal and human sweat and urine. They play important roles in sexual signalling and in marking out territory, although in humans their significance has decreased. In the Russell et al. experiment, pheromones in the sweat acted as zeitgebers, signalling phases of the menstrual cycle and affecting the endogenous menstrual pacemakers so that the cycles of the two women eventually synchronized.

A more elusive infradian rhythm is **seasonal affective disorder** (SAD), when many people report feeling depressed during the winter months. Although this was initially treated with some scepticism, it is now accepted as a genuine clinical syndrome. People with SAD show the classic symptoms of depression – low mood, feelings of hopelessness, loss of interest in normal activities, changes to sleep patterns and so on. Evidence in favour of SAD as a 'real' syndrome is that for some people with SAD, exposure to bright light in the morning can be an effective treatment. We have already seen that light is a major zeitgeber for synchronizing biological rhythms such as sleep and waking, and we shall see later that the effects of light involve the hormone **melatonin**. Melatonin is found throughout the body, including the brain. It shows a circadian rhythm, decreasing during the day and increasing during the night, and is a part of the brain's sleep–waking systems. People with SAD may have some disturbance of the melatonin system that shows itself as day length shortens with the onset of winter. Bright light in the morning may act to resynchronize biological rhythms with the outside world. We have a closer look at SAD at the end of this chapter.

Ultradian rhythms

These are biological rhythms that have more than one complete cycle in 24 hours. The best example is the patterning of the different stages of sleep.

We deal with sleep in detail in Chapter 3. In outline, we have two basic forms of sleep, **rapid eye movement** (REM) and **non-rapid eye movement** (NREM). In phases of REM, rapid movements of the eye are seen and the extremities of legs and arms twitch (REM is particularly obvious in sleeping cats and dogs). NREM sleep is altogether quieter with few outward signs except for the fact that the person is peacefully asleep. When we first fall asleep, we enter a light stage of NREM, then gradually fall more deeply asleep. After some time in the deeper stages of NREM, sleep lightens, and we shift into a phase of REM. This lasts for about 15 minutes, then we move back into the light stages of NREM, and the pattern repeats itself. One cycle of NREM and REM sleep takes about 90 minutes, so we pass through about five cycles during each night of sleep; the patterning of REM and NREM sleep is therefore an ultradian rhythm. The intricate patterning is controlling through sophisticated interactions between the brain centres of arousal outlined in Chapter 1 and further discussed in Chapter 3.

Psychology as science → **Non-rapid eye movement sleep and slow wave sleep**

Confusingly, there are two conventions used in referring to the different types of sleep. Rapid eye movement or REM is used in both. The other type of sleep can be referred to as non-rapid eye movement (NREM) sleep, or **slow wave sleep** (SWS). Across a range of text-books, you will find roughly half follow one system and half the other. Technically, in relation to human sleep, NREM is the more accurate term. Not all the stages of sleep outside the stage of REM (see Chapter 3) actually involve recognizable slow waves, and so are more accurately called non-REM sleep. However, research into sleep has often used REM and SWS. This is particularly important in an evolutionary context, where some animals, for example reptiles, insects, aquatic mammals, only show one type of sleep, which seems to be the equivalent of human SWS. If there is only one type of sleep, it makes no sense to call it NREM as there is no REM phase to compare it with. In this book, I have adopted the REM/NREM convention, but if you do consult other texts, remember that SWS and NREM are often referred to interchangeably. The classification of sleep stages is further discussed in the Chapter 3.

Other examples of ultradian rhythms are less obvious. Even before birth, babies show a rest–activity cycle of about 90 minutes, and there are claims that similar rhythms of rest–activity and drowsiness–alertness across the 24-hour day can be identified in adults (Friedman and Fisher, 1967). It is far more difficult to identify such rhythms as they are less clear-cut than the obvious alternation between REM and NREM sleep.

Ultradian rhythms oscillate too frequently for there to be a systematic role for exogenous environmental zeitgebers, as there are none that change equally frequently and consistently. Therefore it can be argued that ultradian rhythms are almost certainly the expression of endogenous pacemakers, or body clocks, located in the brain. In Chapter 3, we look in detail at the body clocks involved in the control of the REM and NREM ultradian rhythm of sleep.

◉ Endogenous pacemakers

The different types of biological rhythm described above all have one thing in common – rhythmic activity. This activity persists in free-running studies in the laboratory, even if it may not be perfectly synchronized with the outside world. So these brain centres must be able to generate rhythmic activity entirely on their own. We shall use the best-known example of an endogenous pacemaker to illustrate how these rhythms are generated and how they can interact with zeitgebers.

The suprachiasmatic nucleus

A nucleus in the brain is a collection of the cell bodies of neurons, clustered together and tightly packed. The hypothalamus (mentioned above in relation to the pituitary gland) is a brain structure close to the ventral (bottom) surface of the brain. It is made up of a number of distinct nuclei. Many of these centres in the hypothalamus have key functions in relation to physiological functions of the body, such as feeding and drinking behaviour, and controlling the release of hormones from the pituitary gland.

The **suprachiasmatic nucleus** (SCN) is also part of the hypothalamus. It is tiny in comparison with other parts of the brain, being made up of about 10,000 neuronal cell bodies. In 1972 it was shown that lesions (damage) to the SCN had dramatic effects on biological rhythms (Stephan and Zucker, 1972). In particular, the circadian pattern of release of various hormones, such as coricosterone (a hormone linked to our stress response), was disrupted. In addition, the circadian patterns seen in behaviours such as eating and drinking in rats were abolished.

These results showed that the SCN has a key role in the control of circadian rhythms. More importantly, in relation to the topics in this book, it was also shown that SCN lesions disrupted the circadian rhythm of sleep. Although the amount of sleep and the ultradian rhythm of REM and NREM were generally unaffected, sleep and waking became disconnected from the external light–dark cycle and were desynchronized from the onset of light and dark.

A central question was, how does the tiny SCN, with its 10,000 neurons, manage to control a range of circadian rhythms? The key is that they have their own inbuilt rhythm. Studies demonstrated that if the SCN is left in the brain but isolated by cutting all its connections (pathways) to other brain structures, its neurons retain a circadian rhythmic firing pattern. This is also seen if SCN neurons are extracted and kept alive in the laboratory – they still show a circadian pattern of firing, being more active during the daylight phase and less active during the dark phase as they would have been in the intact animal.

The role of the SCN as the main pacemaker for circadian rhythms was further demonstrated in a series of transplantation studies using a strain of hamsters that had an abnormal circadian rhythm of 20 hours rather than 24. SCN neurons from these abnormal hamsters were transplanted into the brains of normal hamsters. The main finding was that the circadian rhythm of the hamsters receiving the transplanted SCN neurons changed to 20 hours from the normal 24, showing the transplanted SCN neurons had imposed their natural pattern onto the recipient's brain. Final confirmation came when the reverse experiment was done. SCN neurons from normal hamsters with a circadian pattern of 24 hours were transplanted into the brains of the 'abnormal' hamsters. Rather than their 20-hour rhythm, the recipient hamsters changed to a circadian rhythm of 24 hours (Morgan, 1995).

So SCN neurons function as the key circadian pacemaker in the brain. They can do this as they have an inbuilt, genetic, or intrinsic circadian firing pattern, and through their connections to other brain structures, they can impose this circadian rhythm on a wide variety of physiological and behavioural processes. We shall see later how the SCN interacts with our visual system to ensure that the circadian sleep–waking cycle is synchronized with the day–night cycle. We should also remember that there are ultradian and infradian rhythms, and these would require their own endogenous pacemakers, or body clocks. So while we know a great deal about the SCN, there are many other brain centres involved in the control of biological rhythms.

⊙ Disrupting biological rhythms

Animals live their lives in natural surroundings, with biological rhythms synchronized to the natural rhythms of light and dark, the movement of the tides, day length, temperature and so on. Humans similarly have a complex network of endogenous pacemakers controlling their biological rhythms, but our social and cultural development has allowed us to break up the normal synchronization with the external world. In some cases, this is due to our colonization of extreme environments. The Inuit, or Eskimos, live in Arctic areas that have months of virtually total night followed by months of virtually total day. However, they still tend to keep to regular patterns of sleeping and waking. This shows that we can respond to zeitgebers other than light and dark. These could include social habits, meal patterns and rhythms of work and recreation.

In this sense, the Inuit do not have disrupted biological rhythms as they are keeping in tune with their intrinsic biological pacemakers. Disruption occurs when we try to act against our inbuilt pacemakers. There are two key areas where this has happened; shiftwork and international jet travel.

Shiftwork

Electric light was invented by Edison in the nineteenth century, and its effects cannot be exaggerated. Before electric lighting, only the rich could afford the candles that would allow social and work life to continue after dark. The poor lived in the same way as animals, in the sense that they operated according to the natural rhythms of light and dark; activity would begin with sunrise and end with nightfall. Electric light changed all that, particularly when it became widespread through the early years of the twentieth century. By the 1950s, we could effectively work and play for 24 hours a day, a complete and rapid transformation of modern societies.

This has had general effects. It is estimated that we now sleep for around 1.5 hours less each night than we did 100 years ago (7.5 hours versus 9 hours), suggesting that mild sleep deprivation could now be quite widespread (Coren, 1996). It also means that we can be active at times when our endogenous pacemakers, or body clocks, are trying to impose rest and sleep. We all experience this at some time, perhaps due to an all-night party or the need to revise late into the evening for important examinations. Usually it is only for a short period and we recover quickly. However, we have also developed more systematic ways to disrupt biological rhythms.

Henry Ford, the pioneer of mass car production, first set up a car assembly line that could operate 24 hours a day in 1914. He could only do this with the required technology, generation of electricity, and round-the-clock availability of good electric lighting. Such industrial production techniques rapidly spread as consumer demand increased, also stimulated by the need for increased output of weapons and machinery during the First and Second World Wars.

However, a problem for continuous mass production is that workers have to do it, and some of them have to work at times when their body clock is telling them it is time to rest and sleep. Besides industrial workers, of course, this includes doctors, nurses and air traffic controllers, for example. No one can work 24 hours a day, so from the earliest car assembly lines, shiftwork has been a regular feature of such jobs. Classically, shifts have been organized on an eight-hour pattern; midnight to 8am, 8am to 4pm, 4pm to midnight. Workers would stay on one shift for, say, a week, then rotate. The standard pattern was to rotate backwards, so one week on midnight to 8am was followed by a week on 4pm to midnight, then a week on 8am to 4pm. It has been estimated that 1 in 5 of American workers do shiftwork.

From our knowledge of biological rhythms and the interaction between endogenous body clocks and exogenous zeitgebers, we can predict the effects. The whole point of endogenous rhythms is to synchronize the body's physiological processes with the outside world. This ensures that we have the energy and arousal to be alert and active during the day, while imposing sleep and recuperation during the night (remember, as we saw in Chapter 1, sleep is not a passive state that happens when nothing much is going on, but an active state imposed on the brain). Put simply, this means that when you are trying to revise at 2am in the morning, your body clock is trying to impose sleep on the brain; you are desynchronizing the endogenous pacemakers from the most influential external zeitgeber, light, by trying to be active and alert at the wrong time.

Thinking scientifically → **The effects of shiftwork**

Now think of someone on the midnight to 8am shift. For night after night, they are trying to perform often complex behaviours at times when their brain is trying to sleep. Obviously it can be done, as many thousands of people do it, but in doing so, they are disrupting their biological rhythms and there are significant costs.

Some of the most devastating accidents of modern times have been linked to night shiftworkers taking the wrong decisions in the early morning (2am to 4am). These include the Chernobyl nuclear power plant explosion and the incident at the Three Mile Island nuclear plant in the USA, where meltdown was only just avoided. Note that the early morning is when the sleep drive is strongest and sleepiness is most likely to impair judgement. More systematic studies have shown that nurses on night shift are far more likely to have car accidents (Gold et al., 1992), and that long periods of shiftwork are associated with an increased risk of heart disease and breast cancer (Davis et al., 2001).

Accidents and major health problems are dramatic, but only the tip of the iceberg. Shiftworkers regularly report higher levels of stress, minor health problems and sleeping difficulties (Coren, 1996). Night shiftworkers are trying to sleep in the daytime, against their natural biological rhythm. They also have to cope with increased levels of noise, daylight itself, and the natural inclination to join in family and social events. So besides the disruption of biological rhythms caused by shiftwork, they may also be sleep deprived.

Although these are difficult areas for researchers to do carefully controlled studies, it is critical that they are carried out. Unlike many laboratory studies, with their lack of ecological validity, research into real-life shiftwork has direct implications and applications for people living lives in the real world.

As research into the role of endogenous pacemakers increased, find-ings could be applied to the harmful effects of shiftwork. One of the pioneers of this area was Charles Czeisler. By the 1970s, it was clear that people suffered harmful consequences from shiftwork and jet lag. In fact, the study of jet lag produced one of the key findings. London time is about five hours ahead of New York time. So when you fly east–west from London to New York, a trip taking about six hours, leaving at 12 noon means that, with the time difference, you arrive in New York at about 1pm local time although your body thinks it is 6pm. This desyn-chronization of endogenous pacemakers from exogenous zeitgebers leads to the symptoms of jet lag. The same dislocation happens when you fly west–east, New York to London, except that leaving New York at 12 noon local time (5pm London time) means that you arrive in London at 11pm local time, although your body clock thinks it is five hours earlier – 6pm. These two experiences are termed phase delay and phase advance:

- **phase delay**: Flying east–west means that when you arrive, your body clock, the endogenous pacemaker, is ahead of local time and has to 'wait' for zeitgebers to catch up.
- **phase advance**: West–east travel leads to the opposite situation, with the pacemaker behind local time, and has to catch up.

It is a common observation that jet lag is significantly less severe when travelling east–west than travelling west–east, suggesting that our endogenous pacemakers find it easier to adjust by phase delay than by phase advance.

Thinking scientifically → Czeisler and shift rotation

Czeisler applied this observation to shiftwork. By tradition, workers moved through the three eight-hour classic shifts backwards; a week, say, on 4pm to midnight, then a week on 8am to 4pm, then a week on midnight to 8am. Czeisler noted that adjusting to each new shift was effectively phase advance, as the endogenous pacemaker is constantly ahead of real time. He reasoned that moving to a system of phase delay, that is, having workers move forward at each shift change (4pm to midnight, then midnight to 8am, then 8am to 4pm), would help the workers adjust in the same way that jet lag is less after phase delay than after phase advance.

Czeisler also considered the time it takes for the body clock to adjust to a new set of zeitgebers, in particular the light–dark cycle. Although there are considerable individual differences, it can take days for full adjustment to occur. A shift rotation of one week means that many workers will be in a constant state of desynchronization, with body clocks never fully adjusted to light and dark. So he also suggested extending the time on any particular shift rotation.

In 1982, Czeisler tested his ideas at a Utah chemical plant, where workers were on a traditional backwards rotation of eight-hour shifts changing every week. They reported high levels of stress and health problems. The change to a forwards shift rotation every 21 days had dramatic effects. After nine months on this schedule, workers reported lower levels of stress and fewer health problems. They were sleeping better, and productivity at the plant increased (Czeisler et al., 1982). A second study found similar results. Changing Philadelphia police officers from a backwards shift rotation to a forwards rotation and extending time on shift to 18 days produced significantly less stress, less sleeping on the job, and a 40% reduction in accidents while working (Coren, 1996).

Findings of these and similar studies support the harmful effects of disrupting biological rhythms. So that we can operate effectively, our endogenous pacemakers are usually synchronized with the outside world through the effect of exogenous zeitgebers, in particular the natural cycles of light and dark. Shiftwork disrupts this normal arrangement. Our body clock is designed to prepare the body for arousal and alertness during the day, and for rest and sleep at night. When we work at night-time, we are going against our body's physiological inclinations. Over time, our body clock can readjust to the new schedule, but while it is adjusting, performance is likely to be impaired. Research has also shown that repeated cycles of readjustment, as with long periods of shiftwork, can lead to stress, serious health problems, and poor work performance.

Changes such as those introduced by Czeisler reduce the effects of shiftwork but do not eliminate them. We have inherited endogenous pacemakers designed to work with exogenous zeitgebers in a particular way, and if we artificially disrupt biological rhythms, there will be a price to pay.

Before looking at the related problem of jet lag, there are alternative ideas on how the harmful effects of shiftwork might be reduced:

- *Planned naps (short periods of sleep) during work hours:* These can reduce stress and improve performance, but are hard to organize and control (Sack et al., 2007). There is a popular view that 'power napping' during the day can be effective even in non-shiftwork. This gains some support from findings that there are ultradian variations in arousal during the day, with a dip in alertness in the early afternoon.
- *Non-rotating shiftwork:* Employees select which of the three eight-hour shifts they want to work and stay on that shift. This allows circadian rhythms to adjust to external zeitgebers as well as they possibly can. Phillips et al. (1991) found this to be an effective remedy for the problems of shiftwork in a study with a Kentucky

police force. However, although this might look like an ideal solution, there can be a problem with finding enough employees prepared to work permanent night shifts.

An indirect help with shiftwork is to ensure that night workers have improved sleep in the daytime. Small changes such as avoiding bright light and keeping the bedroom as dark and quiet as possible can be effective, but can be difficult to implement as the rest of the noisy world is simultaneously going about its business.

Jet lag

Many people experience jet lag after long flights either east–west or west–east. It is caused by travelling through time zones – London is five hours ahead of New York and eight hours ahead of San Francisco. Making flights of the same length but travelling north to south does not lead to jet lag; the key difference is that with north–south flights, you stay in the same time zone. As outlined above, the speed of jet travel means that our endogenous pacemakers do not have time to adjust to the time difference. Travelling from London at midday, you arrive in New York at about 1pm local time, although your body clock thinks it is about 6pm. This is, of course, a phenomenon of jet travel. Making the same trip by boat gives the body clock time to gradually adjust to the different time zones.

There can be individual differences in the pattern of jet lag symptoms, but usually they include tiredness, sleepiness, loss of concentration, increased anxiety and depression, and sometimes irritability. Some people recover quickly, within a few hours, but for others the symptoms can persist for days. As we saw above, symptoms are usually worse travelling west–east (phase advance) than from east–west. A study on American servicemen showed that they took on average eight days to adjust after travelling from the USA to Germany (west–east), but only three days when travelling back to the USA (east–west). In a less controlled study, Recht et al. (1995) looked at the results of American baseball teams over a three-year period. Teams travelling east–west before a game won on average 44% of games, but when travelling west–east, they won only 37%, a difference that was statistically significant. The conclusion was that the more severe effects of jet lag after west–east trips affected performance. However, the relative abilities of the different teams was not controlled for, although it was assumed that over a three-year period, any differences would have evened out.

One group who are exposed to the long-term effects of jet lag are aircrew – pilots and cabin staff. Several studies have shown that over weeks and months, the effects become far more severe. For instance, Cho et al. (2000) showed that aircrew on regular long-haul flights had raised levels of the stress hormone **cortisol**, and performed less well than control participants on tests of memory. In a further study from the same research group (Cho, 2001), female aircrew with several years of long-haul experience did worse that aircrew with less experience on reaction time and memory tests. They also had elevated cortisol levels, and brain scans showed shrinkage of structures in the temporal lobes of the brain. Incidentally, it is known that raised levels of cortisol in the bloodstream, often associated with high levels of stress, can have toxic effects on neurons in the hippocampus (MacEwen, 2000).

There is no direct evidence that disruption of biological rhythms caused the effects observed in these experiments. However, the use of appropriate control groups and our knowledge of the short-term effects of jet lag make it a justifiable conclusion. Repeated exposure to the desynchronization of biological rhythms from exogenous zeitgebers has serious effects on physiological and cognitive processes. This is supported by the findings of increased risk of heart disease and cancer from long-term shiftwork mentioned earlier.

Jet travel is now an established part of everyday life, although most of us will experience it only once or twice year, if we are lucky. Aircrew and those involved in international business use it regularly and have to cope with the repeated stress of jet lag. One important strand of research is aimed at finding ways of reducing the effects of jet lag.

Coping with jet lag

There are a number of variables that affect the severity of jet lag. These include, as we have seen, the direction of travel, whether east–west or west–east. Also important are the distance travelled, that is, the number of time zones crossed, and it's also clear that people differ in their vulnerability to jet lag. One aspect of these individual differences might be age, as studies have shown that the severity of jet lag decreases the older you are.

Besides these natural variables, there are some adjustments an individual can make that have been shown to reduce jet lag (Coren, 1996). Perhaps the most important is to synchronize with the local zeitgebers as soon as you arrive. This means that if you arrive in the evening, then prepare for sleep, and if you arrive in the daytime, then stay awake and alert. Given that we know that early morning daylight is an important zeitgeber for synchronizing biological rhythms, it also helps to wake in the early morning at your destination and go out into the sunlight.

If you are one of those people who suffer only mild jet lag, these adjustments should help and symptoms should not last more than a day or so. If you are sensitive to the effects of jet lag, again these adjustments would help, but symptoms may still last for several days. Because the symptoms can be unpleasant, and even though we know that everyone will readjust eventually, research has explored the use of drugs to help reduce jet lag. In particular the hormone melatonin has been studied. As we shall see in Chapter 3, melatonin plays an important role in the brain mechanisms underlying biological rhythms. Levels of melatonin in the brain are reduced by sunlight and increase during darkness. In principle, altering levels of melatonin artificially should affect biological rhythms, and there are some studies demonstrating that this can be useful in coping with jet lag. Arendt et al. (1987) found that melatonin taken during the evening at the destination produces a more rapid adjustment of circadian rhythms and synchronizes them with local zeitgebers. Supporting these findings, Beaumont et al. (2004) gave their participants melatonin in the evening for three days before travel and for five days after arrival at their destination. They found that this significantly reduced the symptoms of jet lag.

Seasonal affective disorder (SAD) and biological rhythms

SAD, besides being an infradian rhythm, is also thought to reflect a subtle disruption of biological rhythms. We have seen that melatonin can help in adjustments to the disruption of biological rhythms caused by jet lag. If SAD is also related to problems with the control of biological rhythms, might directly manipulating melatonin levels help? Bright light treatment in the early morning can help some people with SAD, and we know that light has a direct effect on brain melatonin levels. So, logically, it would seem that altering melatonin levels directly should help, but the problem is the complexity of the control of biological rhythms. Doses of melatonin can 'shift' circadian rhythms, but in different ways at different times. Taken in the morning, it can phase delay rhythms, but taken in the evening, it can phase advance rhythms – remember, melatonin levels increase during the hours of darkness and decrease during daylight. So additional melatonin medication will have different effects at different times. Because of this complexity, effective treatments for SAD using melatonin have so far been elusive.

Psychology as science → **Does SAD exist?**

SAD still is not fully accepted as a clinical disorder, but what would help convince sceptics would be the identification of the causes of the disorder. Low mood affects many people during the winter months, strongly suggesting that day length (light) and/or temperature may play a role. If day length was the crucial variable, then we can make a straightforward prediction that SAD should vary with day length, and therefore vary with how far north on the globe people live. We grade north versus south using measures of latitude, which varies from $+90^0$ at the Arctic, 0^0 at the equator, and -90^0 at the Antarctic. London, for instance, is at about 50^0 of latitude.

Days become shorter the further north we live, that is, at greater degrees of latitude. Mersch et al. (1999) reviewed all the available studies of SAD at that time and found that the frequency of SAD in the USA did correlate with latitude. However, studies carried out in Europe did not find such a correlation. How do we explain this contradiction? What are the differences between the USA and Europe that might explain it?

- People in the USA are in general more aware of psychological health and conditions such as SAD. They might be more prepared to describe such symptoms. In Europe, social and cultural values might act against admitting conditions such as depression.
- There might be differences between areas at the same latitude (day length) in the USA and Europe; for instance, climate. Madrid and New York are roughly at the same latitude, but have very different climates. New York suffers more dramatic changes in weather, with greater extremes of hot and cold than Madrid. This may have unpredictable effects on mood.
- The populations of the USA and Europe may have subtle genetic differences that influence vulnerability to SAD.

The aim of the scientific approach in psychology is to identify the key variables. However, in this area of research, it is virtually impossible to do controlled experiments, systematically manipulating the independent variable. Greater reliance is placed on the use of **correlations**. However, correlations can only show an association, and do not identify cause-and-effect relationships. For instance, personality variables may explain some of the characteristics of SAD. Winter is a gloomy dark time. People prone to depression might *expect* to feel more depressed as the days get shorter, especially if they are aware of SAD as a syndrome. So research into SAD needs to take into account social, cultural and personality variables as well as factors such as day length.

Summary

- All living organisms demonstrate biological rhythms of some sort. These are divided into circadian, infradian and ultradian rhythms.
- Studies of free-running circadian rhythms in animals and humans show that internal body clocks (endogenous pacemakers) can maintain body rhythms but are not perfectly accurate. External stimuli, such as light onset, act as zeitgebers and synchronize biological rhythms with the outside world.
- Some biological rhythms, such as the menstrual cycle and the alternation of REM and NREM sleep during the night, rely far more on internal body clocks than zeitgebers.
- There are many endogenous pacemakers to control over 100 biological rhythms in complex animals. The most studied has been the suprachiasmatic nucleus (SCN) in the hypothalamus. Neurons that make up the SCN have their own intrinsic or built-in rhythmic activity.
- Both shiftwork and jet travel can disrupt biological rhythms, especially the circadian sleep–waking cycle. Disruption can lead to psychological ill health, physical illness and problems of absenteeism and lowered productivity.
- Using techniques based on our knowledge of endogenous pacemakers and their interaction with zeitgebers, the negative effects of shiftwork and jet lag can be reduced.
- Seasonal affective disorder (SAD) is an infradian circannual rhythm in which some people suffer lethargy and depression with the onset of winter. It may have an evolutionary link to the preparations for hibernation still seen in animals such as squirrels and bears. Although some people respond to treatment with bright light, there is no simple association with day length.

Chapter 3

Sleep

👁 Introduction

The experience of sleep has stimulated many of the basic questions of consciousness and awareness. There is no doubt that we are unconscious through much of a night's sleep, but how about dreams? In these, we are apparently aware and conscious, but with no sense that it is 'we' who are dreaming. It seems to be a state of awareness or primary consciousness, rather than the state of higher consciousness and self-awareness associated with waking. The study of sleep may help unpack some of the issues surrounding consciousness.

We have already covered some aspects of sleep. The sleep–waking cycle is a circadian biological rhythm. During a night's sleep, the alternation between periods of rapid eye movement (REM) and non-rapid eye movement (NREM) sleep represents an ultradian biological rhythm. However, there are many major questions to be answered.

About the only aspect of sleep that researchers can agree on is that humans seem to need a lot of it. We spend roughly one-third of our lives asleep, amounting to some 25 years if you are lucky. It would seem obvious that such a phenomenon must have important physiological and maybe psychological functions. But, as we shall see, there is still no agreement on what these functions might be. There are many hypotheses, ranging from whether animals are predators or prey, down to the activity of neurons in the brain. In this chapter, we review some of the characteristics of sleep across the animal kingdom and consider some of the major theories as to why sleep evolved and what its functions might be.

In this chapter, we will cover:
- Stages of sleep
- Brain mechanisms of REM and NREM sleep
- Functions of sleep
- Evolutionary/ecological theories of sleep
- Contemporary evolutionary/ecological approaches
- Restoration theories of sleep
- Sleep and learning
- Sleep across the life span

Psychology as science → **The sleep laboratory**

We shall start by briefly reviewing some of the methods used in sleep research. In Chapter 1 we saw how the electroencephalograph (EEG) can be used as an index of the brain state of general arousal or activation. The EEG was introduced by Hans Berger (1929), who identified some of its basic characteristics such as synchronized and desynchronized patterns, and alpha and beta waves. Today the EEG remains a key technology in the study of sleep, although these days it is usually just one part of the sleep laboratory. Later in the chapter we shall see that many of the early observations on sleep were based on case studies and sometimes just casual observation. The modern sleep laboratory for research into human sleep operates under far more controlled conditions. Besides the EEG, many other physiological functions will be measured, including eye movements, levels of hormones in the blood stream and muscle activity. The simultaneous recording of these physiological measures is referred to as **polysomnography**. There will also be facilities for testing memory and attention and other cognitive processes. Sleep laboratories are also set up so that participants can be studied constantly for days at a time.

However, it must also be remembered that the sleep laboratory is an artificial environment, and sleep phenomena are likely to be different to sleep in natural surroundings. For instance, early research using the sleep laboratory to investigate dreams found that dream imagery often included aspects of the laboratory itself. To try and control this, participants are familiarized with the laboratory over several days before serious recording begins.

◉ Stages of sleep

Early research

Although Loomis (1937) had first used the EEG to investigate brain activity during sleep, the first systematic sleep laboratory was set up by Nathaniel Kleitman and in the 1950s this laboratory made some of the most exciting discoveries on the nature and characteristics of sleep. Eugene Aserinsky, one of Kleitman's students, was the first to record a continuous EEG throughout a night's sleep (at this time no one suspected that different brain states might occur during sleep), initially on his young son but then more systematically on a number of adult participants. In 1953, Aserinsky and Kleitman published their dramatic findings. They demonstrated conclusively that there were at least two different patterns of sleep. After falling asleep, a person's EEG gradually becomes synchronized and the waves become slower and larger (see Figure 3.1). After about 70 minutes though, the EEG recording changes to the arousal pattern; it becomes desynchronized with low amplitude fast activity, a pattern resembling the aroused, waking EEG. This is accompanied by rapid movements of the eyes and a loss of muscle tone so that the person is effectively paralysed. However, there may be twitching movements of the fingers and toes (particularly obvious in sleeping cats and dogs).

Aserinsky and Kleitman called this unusual sleep pattern rapid eye movement (REM) sleep. Despite the arousal pattern of the EEG, the person is hard to awake, that is, is deeply asleep; so a more old-fashioned term for this type of sleep is **paradoxical sleep**, as an aroused EEG is combined with behavioural sleep. After 20–30 minutes in REM, the EEG changes back to the synchronized pattern (NREM sleep) with increasingly slow, large waves. Throughout a night's sleep, this alternation of different types of sleep continues, and in a night's sleep, you might have four or five episodes of REM sleep.

Aserinsky and Kleitman followed up these initial findings, working particularly with William Dement (Dement and Kleitman, 1957), and were able to provide a detailed account of the ultradian rhythm of sleep stages and the association between REM and dreaming. Incidentally, Dement originally intended to train as a psychoanalyst and was particularly fond of the writings of Freud on dreams.

The different stages of sleep

The EEG has been fundamental in defining states of awareness and in particular the stages of sleep. You will recall that EEG patterns can be synchronized or desynchronized, and if synchronized they can be defined in terms of the frequency (cycles per second or herz, Hz) and amplitude (size of the waves). NREM sleep, in particular, is defined by these EEG characteristics (see Figure 3.1). These are the stages of NREM sleep:

- *Stage 1:* Relaxed wakefulness is characterized by **alpha waves**, in which the EEG is synchronized with small waves at a frequency of between 8–12 Hz. The drowsy person has an EEG dominated by **theta waves**. Again these are smallish waves but the frequency is slower at between 4–7 Hz. This is counted as the first stage of NREM sleep, although it more properly represents a drowsy stage between waking and sleep.
- *Stage 2:* It is in stage 2 of NREM sleep that the person is properly asleep, with the EEG still showing theta waves of higher amplitude than in stage 1. In this stage, we also see sleep spindles in the EEG – short bursts of roughly half a second of high frequency (12–15 Hz) activity.
- *Stage 3:* Stage 3 of NREM sleep sees the appearance of **delta waves** – high amplitude slow waves with a frequency of 1–4 Hz. Sleep spindles are less frequent.
- *Stage 4:* In stage 4 NREM sleep, the person is most deeply asleep and the EEG is dominated by delta waves.

Psychology as science → **NREM sleep and slow wave sleep (SWS)**

In Chapter 2, we discussed the different systems used by researchers to describe the various stages of sleep, with NREM and SWS used as virtual synonyms. To resolve these issues, the American Academy of Sleep Medicine (2005) has introduced a more systematic system. NREM sleep is divided into three stages – N1, N2 and N3:

- *N1* is equivalent to stage 1 NREM, when the person is in relaxed wakefulness, between sleeping and waking. There may be loss of conscious awareness and the EEG is dominated by alpha waves.
- *N2* is equivalent to stage 2 NREM, when the person is fully asleep and the EEG is dominated by theta waves along with the occurrence of sleep spindles.
- *N3* is deep slow wave sleep, with the EEG showing at least 20% delta waves. It therefore covers both stages 3 and 4 NREM. N3 NREM is the equivalent of SWS.

This system has not yet come into widespread use, but is likely to become more popular over the coming years. However, it is not without its critics. Comparisons with the previous system (Rechtschaffen and Kales, 1968) have found that the new system produces scores for various aspects of sleep that are not highly correlated with scores from the earlier system (Novelli et al., 2009). These discrepancies will have to be resolved. For the moment, we shall stay with the classic four stages of NREM sleep, remembering that only stages 3 and 4 represent slow wave sleep.

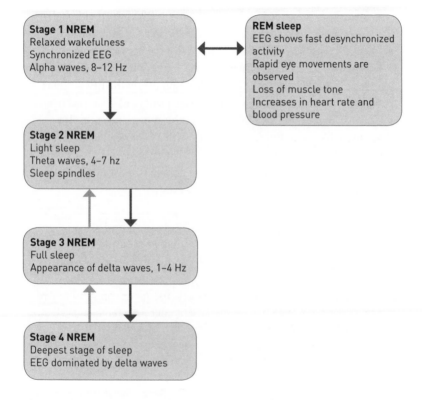

Figure 3.1 Stages of sleep

The progression from drowsiness to stage 4 NREM takes about 75 minutes. At that point, sleep lightens and we move back up into stage 2 NREM. It is at this stage that we move into the fifth stage of sleep, REM sleep. The EEG recording shows fast desynchronized activity, rapid eye movements are observed and there is a loss of muscle tone. Other physiological characteristics of REM sleep include increases in heart rate and blood pressure, and there may be penile erections in males and an increase in vaginal blood flow in females.

After 15–20 minutes in REM, the person moves back into stage 2 NREM and repeats the progression down to stage 4 NREM. This cycle of NREM alternating with phases of REM takes about 90 minutes and so we have four or five cycles during a night's sleep (Figure 3.1). Towards morning we tend to spend longer in the lighter stages 2 and 3 NREM, and we also spend longer in REM sleep. Stage 4 NREM (deep SWS) virtually disappears towards morning.

REM and dreaming

Yet another pioneering discovery by Kleitman's group was the association between REM sleep and dreaming (Dement and Kleitman, 1957). When their participants were woken during REM sleep, they reported dreaming about 80% of the time. The comparable figure for those woken during NREM sleep was 20%. The researchers also noted differences in the quality of the dreams reported. REM dreams were more intense, and tended to be narrative, with a clear storyline, while NREM dreams tended to be more fragmented and incoherent.

These findings rapidly caught the public's imagination and REM sleep was quickly given a third possible name, that of 'dreaming sleep'. However, there are some problems with this simple equation between REM and dreaming. First, we have already seen that dreams also occur in NREM. Second, when people report dreams, they are reporting a subjective experience; we have no scientific way of recording dreams and dream imagery, and rely completely on the person's verbal description. REM sleep, in contrast, is a physiological state that is clearly defined by distinctive patterns in the EEG and other physiological measures.

REM sleep and dreaming are therefore very different concepts. We will see in Chapter 5 that some theories of dreaming make no reference to REM at all, while others try to explain dreams through the brain mechanisms of REM sleep. However, note that when we are discussing the functions of the different types of sleep, we are concerned with the physiological state known as REM, and not with the dreams that may be associated with it.

◉ Brain mechanisms of REM and NREM sleep

In Chapter 1, we referred briefly to the ascending reticular activating system (ARAS) and the work of Jouvet. The ARAS (see Figure 1.1) has its origin in the brainstem and sends neural pathways throughout the brain, controlling the arousal state of higher brain centres. Jouvet (1969) identified two key centres or nuclei in the brainstem ARAS that seemed to play key roles in sleep. Through a series of lesion and stimulation experiments, Jouvet established that:

- The **locus coeruleus** was important in stimulating and controlling REM sleep. Damage to the locus coeruleus significantly reduced the amount of REM, while electrical stimulation could increase the amount of REM.
- The **raphe nuclei** were important in stimulating and controlling deep NREM (SWS). Lesions to the raphe produced severe insomnia.
- Jouvet also identified two brain neurotransmitters (chemicals that act to allow neural impulses to cross the synapse) that were associated with the locus coeruleus and the raphe nuclei. **Noradrenaline**, released by neurons in the locus coeruleus, promoted the onset of REM, while **serotonin**, released from neurons in the raphe nuclei, promoted deep NREM. Decreases in the activity of serotonin induced by drugs led to a reduction in deep NREM that could be reversed by giving drugs that increased serotonin activity.

Jouvet's work provided the first and most influential model of the brain mechanisms of sleep. He identified the vital role of the ARAS and the nuclei within it in the regulation of sleep and in particular in the ultra-dian rhythm of REM and NREM. Pathways originating in the raphe and the locus coeruleus travel through the brain and lead to the pattern of brain activity characteristic of sleep states.

Subsequent research has built on Jouvet's findings and reveals a more complicated picture, far outside the scope of this book. In brief, other

ARAS centres located close to the locus coeruleus play important roles in REM, and nuclei within the hypothalamus are also critical in the control of REM and NREM. Pathways releasing other neurotransmitters, such as acetylcholine and GABA, have been shown to be part of our sleep control systems. All of which supports a picture of sleep and sleep stages involving a large number of centres (nuclei) within the brain, some of which promote sleep at appropriate times, and some of which inhibit sleep. Others are involved in the transition between the different stages of NREM and REM. Paradoxically, sleep is a highly active and compli-cated brain state, far removed from the early ideas that sleep simply represented the state of the brain when nothing much was happening.

Sleep as a circadian rhythm: body clocks and zeitgebers

We saw in Chapter 2 that the suprachiasmatic nucleus (SCN) is an important body clock controlling the circadian rhythm of sleep and arousal. Its neurons have an inbuilt or endogenous circadian rhythm, but to be perfectly synchronized with zeitgebers such as light onset and to control processes such as sleep and waking, the SCN needs to be part of a brain circuit.

The SCN receives information about the amount of light entering the eye through a pathway branching off from the main visual input pathway running from the retina of the eye to the visual cortex. This branch, the **retinohypothalamic tract**, carries information about the amount of light on the retina directly to the SCN. If it is cut, the synchronization of sleep–waking with the light–dark cycle breaks down, similar to the effects of SCN lesions. This shows how light performs its role as our main zeit-geber in relation to sleep–waking. But what happens beyond the SCN?

The next key structure is the pineal gland. This gland, also found in reptiles and amphibia, secretes the hormone melatonin. In reptiles the pineal gland is located in the brain close to the skull surface and it is directly responsive to light, which inhibits the release of melatonin. In mammals such as humans the pineal is buried deep in the brain and is not directly responsive to light. However, it is connected through neural pathways to the SCN, and it is this pathway that allows melatonin secre-tion from the pineal to be affected by the zeitgeber light.

The SCN responds to light input via the retinohypothalamic tract. It then sends messages to the pineal gland to increase or decrease the release of melatonin. In this way, melatonin release is affected by light onset and by darkness. It increases in darkness, and decreases with light onset. Why is this important?

Melatonin is a hormone that has a range of effects on the brain and the body. It leads to a decrease in body temperature and affects the release of a range of other hormones such as the growth hormone. Some of these effects may act as physiological triggers for the onset of sleep. Melatonin can also have direct effects on the SCN itself, allowing for a role in the synchronization of the sleep–waking cycle. Although yet to be finally demonstrated, it is also possible that melatonin may have a direct action on sleep–waking mechanisms of the brainstem ARAS. These functions of melatonin have led to much research into its use as a treatment for jet lag and seasonal affective disorder, outlined in Chapter 2.

Other pathways from the SCN connect to brain areas known to be involved in the sleep–waking cycle and the different phases of sleep. Together with the ARAS sleep–waking centres, the SCN and the pineal gland form part of an incredibly complex network of structures and pathways. The end result is the ultradian patterning of REM and NREM sleep, and the circadian rhythm of sleep and waking synchronizing with light and dark in the external world. The personal experience of sleep can be very straightforward, and it is easy to forget how hard the brain works to make sure it stays that way.

◉ Functions of sleep

Reference has been made previously to early studies that demonstrated clearly that sleep was a state of awareness imposed on the brain, rather than the state the brain lapses into in the absence of sensory input. The idea that sleep is therefore an active process is now fully accepted, to the extent that we can identify many of the pathways and sleep centres involved. The complex structure of sleep and the mechanisms underlying the different phases of sleep suggest that it must have significant and important functions; otherwise there would seem little reason for such complexity to evolve. The idea that sleep must have important functions is also supported by the very obvious point that we spend a third of our lives sleeping.

It is also relevant that sleep is found throughout the animal kingdom. Even though it can be difficult to identify sleep in animals with simple and primitive nervous systems, such as insects, there is evidence that even these simple creatures show rhythms of rest and activity. Further up the animal kingdom, reptiles (for example snakes and lizards) and amphibians (for example frogs and newts) also show rhythmic patterns of rest and activity, even though their brains are relatively primitive compared to mammals. Electrical recording has also been used to identify what looks like the slow wave stages of NREM sleep in such animals (Rattenborg et al., 2009). Although there is still much debate as to whether these animals show genuine sleep, it is indisputable that the most evolved and advanced animal groups, the mammals and birds, all show rhythms of sleep and waking. As we shall see, the amount and patterning of the different phases and stages of sleep vary greatly between different species, but the key observation is that all species of mammal and bird studied sleep.

In many cases, animals go to extraordinary lengths in order to sleep; wildebeest, for instance, will sleep on the open plains of Africa completely exposed to predators. Dolphins are sea-dwelling mammals who need to come to the surface occasionally to breathe; complete sleep would therefore put them in danger of drowning, and so they have evolved the bizarre strategy of sleeping with only one half of the brain at a time. Thus each half of the brain has periods of sleep, during which the awake half can maintain a degree of alertness.

Thinking scientifically → **The puzzle of sleep in dolphins**

Dolphin sleep is an excellent example of why sleep is so fascinating and yet so difficult to understand. John Lilly (1964) was the first to make systematic observations of sleep in captive dolphins, and was the first to notice that dolphins often sleep with one eye closed. Subsequent research by Serafetinides et al. (1972) and Mukhametov et al. (1977) involved developing techniques for EEG recording from free-swimming dolphins and their relatives (dolphins are in a mammalian group called the cetaceans: this also includes porpoises and the Beluga whale. All seem to have the same sleep characteristics).

The first recording attempts involved simply inserting electrodes into the blubber above the skull. Later, a wire harness technique was devised that allowed more reliable recording, and this is now combined with telemetry (meaning that wire connections between dolphin and recording apparatus were not necessary) to allow distance recording in free-swimming dolphins, although they are usually still held in large enclosures. Science has a way of solving problems.

It turns out that dolphin sleep is very special:

- Dolphins show only NREM sleep; they do not appear to have REM sleep
- NREM sleep is usually recorded only from one hemisphere of the brain at a time, in episodes of around 40 minutes, with about five episodes in 24 hours. The hemisphere involved alternates regularly
- While one hemisphere shows unilateral (one-sided) NREM, the other hemisphere usually shows an aroused EEG pattern
- Unilateral NREM is often associated with closure of the eye on the opposite side and opening of the eye on the same side. Control of eye opening is by the opposite side of the brain, so eye closure is linked to the sleeping hemisphere and eye opening with the aroused hemisphere.

This unique pattern of sleeping is almost certainly related to the dolphin's aquatic environment. They need to swim continually and also to be constantly alert for predators, debris in the sea or river and so on. Keeping one hemisphere constantly aroused and alert, with one eye open to scan the environment, may be an adaptation to their ecological niche (Lyamin et al., 2008). This interpretation is supported by the observation that some birds also show unilateral eye opening during sleep (Rattenborg et al., 2009); birds roosting near the edge of flocks tend to show a higher frequency of eye opening, suggesting it is related to detecting danger in the environment. Incidentally, the similarities end there, as birds do show phases of REM as well as NREM sleep.

Sleep in dolphins poses real problems for theories of the functions of sleep. If REM sleep in other animals has important functions, then these functions in dolphins must be organized in very different ways. At present we do not know what these are, although one theory of dreaming does use the dolphin as evidence in its favour.

The fact that sleep is so widespread and the observation that animals will go to such lengths in order to sleep argue powerfully that sleep performs vital functions in all complex animal species. Unfortunately, even after many years of research, we still have no clear idea what these functions are. As we shall see, there are many hypotheses, particularly as the situation has become more complicated since the discovery of the different stages of sleep, REM and NREM. Not only do we have to account for the functions of sleep, but ideally we should also account for the separate functions of REM and NREM sleep.

Fortunately, approaches to explaining the functions of sleep can be divided into two general categories:

1   The **evolutionary/ecological approach** emphasizes the role of sleep in an animal's general lifestyle. It takes into account various characteristics of a species, such as body size, brain size, habitat, sleeping places, whether they are a carnivore or herbivore and so on. One advantage of this approach is that it aims to provide a general explanation for the functions of sleep that could be applied to any species.

2   The **restoration approach** emphasizes the possible restoration functions of sleep. In outline, this is the idea that during sleep our physiological systems can rest and recuperate from the activities of the day, for example we can restore hormone and neurotransmitter levels, and repair any damage to body tissues. Like the ecological accounts, restoration theories can be applied across the animal kingdom.

Besides these two major categories of explanations, there are a number of more restricted hypotheses on the functions of sleep. For example, there is research supporting a role for sleep in cognitive processes such as memory consolidation, an approach that largely focuses on the functions of sleep in humans.

Psychology as science

In retrospect, one mistake made by early theories of the functions of sleep was to assume that there was only one correct theory, and that alternative theories were therefore wrong. It now seems far more likely that a full explanation of the functions of sleep will contain elements of all these approaches. One principle that is often quoted by scientists is 'Occam's razor', or the 'principle of parsimony'. This is the idea that before we construct a complicated explanation or theory, we should see if a simpler one will provide a satisfactory account.

So a single explanation for the functions of sleep across all species is a sensible way to start and reflects the principle of parsimony. However, as findings accumulate, it is often necessary to modify original ideas and accept that the final explanations might be far more complicated than the early ones. This is what has happened as research into the functions of sleep has increased.

◉ Evolutionary/ecological theories of sleep

Sleep is found throughout the animal kingdom, but varies greatly across species in terms of amount and, in some cases, in the patterning of REM and NREM sleep. It is possible by simple observation to identify some general relationships. Large animals, for instance, tend to sleep less than smaller animals; elephants and cows sleep for about four hours a night, while cats sleep for about 15 hours, and small rodents, such as dormice and shrews, may sleep for over 20 hours in 24. Does this mean that the amount of sleep is simply related to body size? The short answer is no. Besides body size, animals also differ in habitat (also known as their ecological niche), brain size, diet and where they actually sleep. These and other ecological factors may influence their sleep patterns. The problem for researchers is to try and untangle the relevant variables, and identify the crucial ones. Life becomes even more complicated if we also want to explain the separate functions of REM and NREM sleep.

Two early studies will give the flavour of the type of research carried out in this area. Zepelin and Rechtschaffen (1974) collected data on sleep time and physiological characteristics of 53 species of mammal. They found a negative correlation between an animal's body size and their total sleep time (total sleep time, TST, includes both REM and NREM). We know that body size is a key index of **basal metabolic rate** (BMR); all the cells in the body are continually active, burning up energy, and BMR is a measure of how active they are and therefore how much energy the body is consuming. BMR is closely linked to overall body size, in that large animals have a lower BMR than small animals. So Zepelin and Rechtschaffen's findings suggest that TST is linked to BMR; the higher an animal's BMR, the more it sleeps. This was one of the first comprehensive studies to show a clear relationship between one characteristic of animals and the amount they slept. Jumping ahead, perhaps you can see how this relationship supports the idea that sleep may have restorative functions. Animals with higher BMRs burn up more energy while awake, but will conserve energy when asleep, which would help restorative processes.

Two years later, Allison and Cicchetti (1976) did a similar study looking at the sleep characteristics in 39 animal species. They focused on whether animals were predators or prey, and found a relationship between the level of danger experienced by an animal in its normal habitat and TST. The two variables were negatively correlated, so that animals in most danger (prey animals) slept less than predators such as lions and leopards. So predator–prey status seemed to be an important variable in determining the amount of sleep.

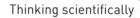

Thinking scientifically

But think about this for a moment. The shrew is a small animal with a high BMR, so it should sleep more. However, it is also a prey animal for larger carnivorous animals and also eagles and hawks, so it should sleep less. Lions are predators and should therefore sleep more, but they are also large mammals with a relatively low BMR and so should sleep less. Even with this simple analysis, we can see that TST will be a function of several variables. We shall see later how complex this type of ecological analysis can become, and how isolating the effects of single variables can be difficult.

Meddis and the safety hypothesis

Around the same time that these first systematic studies were being published, there were also attempts to explain the functions of sleep in more conceptual ways. Meddis (1975) put forward one of the first ecological theories of sleep. He proposed that the key variable was danger and that the simple purpose of sleep was to keep an animal inconspicuous and safe at times when active behaviour was impossible. Diurnal animals, for instance, are adapted to be active during the day and therefore sleep at night. Nocturnal animals are adapted to be active at night, and therefore keep themselves safe during the day by sleeping. An obvious objection to this idea is that it in order to be safe, it would make more sense to be inconspicuous but also to be alert. A counterargument is that an awake animal will always make some movements or sounds so the state of sleep is a way of ensuring that they are completely immobile. A further objection is that the mechanism of sleep, and even the fact that there are two types of sleep (REM and NREM), seems too complex an arrangement simply to ensure that an animal stays still. However, this idea of sleep having a relatively simple function has been recently revived. Rial et al. (2007) propose that sleep has no function apart from ensuring rest, and is, in fact, an evolutionary hangover. This goes against the majority view that sleep does have important, non-trivial functions, but illustrates how difficult it has been to identify these functions.

Webb and the hibernation theory: energy conservation

While Meddis emphasized the safety from danger aspect of sleep, Webb focused on rest and energy conservation. Animals hibernate during the winter in order to reduce energy consumption at times when normal activities such as hunting and foraging are impossible. A key characteristic of hibernation is that the BMR falls to a low level, showing that the animal is using very little of its energy. Night-time for diurnal animals and daytime for nocturnal animals are periods when normal activity is impossible. So, according to Webb's **hibernation theory**, it makes sense for them to rest and conserve their energy resources by sleeping. We have already seen that TST is closely linked to BMR, an index of the usual rate of energy consumption by an animal. So it is advantageous for smaller animals with higher BMRs to sleep for longer, as they are conserving even more of their energy resources (Webb, 1982).

Evidence in favour of this theory of sleep is that energy consumption and BMR decrease significantly during the deeper stages of NREM. Unfortunately for the theory, REM, as we have seen, is a highly active state of the brain, and in fact overall energy consumption by the brain and body is little different to waking levels. So overall energy conservation during sleep is not dramatic, and in fact not very different from simple rest. So we still have the problem of trying to explain why we have a distinctive state of sleep imposed on the brain.

Sleep in mammals: REM and temperature regulation

Research into the functions of sleep has mainly focused on mammals. Mammals include relatively simple animals such as shrews and mice, up to the highly complex primates – monkeys, chimpanzees, orang-utans, gorillas and humans. The distinctive feature of mammals (and also birds) is that they maintain a constant body temperature. This distinguishes them from the reptiles and other so-called 'cold-blooded' animals. In fact, cold-blooded animals are not cold blooded. They do not maintain a constant body temperature, so their temperature varies with the environmental temperature. That is why, if you see snakes and lizards, they are often basking in the sunshine as this raises their body temperature. Increases in body temperature raise the BMR and the animal can be more active.

Another less well-known difference between mammals and reptiles is that although a state of sleep can be identified in reptiles, they do not appear to have REM sleep but only NREM sleep. REM sleep seems to have evolved with mammals and birds and one hypothesis is that REM sleep evolved in association with the maintenance of a constant body temperature. Temperature regulation in NREM is poor and so body temperature falls during NREM sleep. However, regulation is maintained during REM and, so the argument goes, the phases of REM that occur during sleep are critical in maintaining temperature regulation during the night.

The significance of this for Webb's hibernation theory is that when sleep first evolved it was NREM, and, as we have seen, this is associated with energy conservation. So the first and central function of sleep was directly related to energy conservation, supporting Webb's theory. Then, the evolution of mammals introduced the problem of temperature regulation, and REM sleep evolved as an adaptation to the need to maintain a constant body temperature. The cost involved was that sleep was no longer a major source of energy conservation. However, many authors (for example Rial et al., 2007) have pointed out that simple rest can provide the energy conservation that animals need.

⊙ Contemporary evolutionary/ecological approaches

Over the past few decades, information on sleep across the animal kingdom has continued to accumulate. Current approaches can therefore look at a wider range of variables that might influence the amount and patterning of sleep. A good example is the study by Lesku et al. (2006), who collected data on 54 species and analysed the influence of the following variables:

- Body mass
- Brain mass
- Basal metabolic rate (BMR)
- **Sleep exposure index**: this was measured by seeing where the animal slept and how safe this location was. For instance, a rabbit's deep burrow would be a safe place to sleep, while the wildebeest's sleeping site on the open savannah would be seen as a dangerous place to sleep
- **Trophic position**: this refers to an animal's position on the food chain, essentially whether it is a herbivore (surviving on grass, leaves and berries) or a carnivore (meat eater). This can be

significant in several ways. For instance, carnivores are often predators and tend to sleep more than prey animals; herbivores tend to be prey animals, and also have to forage for long periods to obtain the nutrients they need. So they actually have less time available for sleep.

The key findings from Lesku et al.'s study (2006) can be summarized as follows:

- Brain mass was positively correlated with the amount of REM sleep; the larger an animal's brain, in absolute terms, the greater the amount of REM sleep.
- A surprising finding from the study was that BMR was negatively correlated with NREM and TST. This contradicts the findings discussed above that have shown a positive correlation between BMR and TST. One explanation for this discrepancy is that Lesku et al. calculate an animal's BMR in a rather unconventional way. Other studies (for example Savage and West, 2007) support the positive correlation between BMR and TST.
- The sleep exposure index was negatively correlated with the amount of REM sleep. Animals with more dangerous sleeping locations had less REM sleep.
- There was a positive correlation between trophic position and the amount of REM sleep and also TST. Carnivores had more REM sleep and more TST than herbivores.

In a later paper, Lesku et al. (2008) also found that the amount of REM sleep correlated positively with the degree of brain encephalization. This refers to how advanced an animal's brain is in evolutionary terms. A simple measure is to take the ratio of brain size to body size. More advanced animals such as humans and dolphins have a high **encephalization quotient** (EQ), while less advanced animals have a low EQ. Lesku et al. found that the higher an animal's EQ, the more REM sleep it had.

Studies such as these, reviewing the characteristics of animals in relation to their sleep patterns, lead to some general conclusions, but also show how many of the variables interact with each other. We should also note that all these studies are correlational. This means that they can show an association between a particular variable and sleep patterns, but they do not identify a cause-and-effect relationship. So we must be cautious in drawing conclusions.

With that cautionary note in mind, we can draw some general conclusions from research into the evolutionary/ecological approach to the functions of sleep:

- Body size is negatively correlated with sleep time, so that small animals sleep for longer than larger animals.
- Although findings are not entirely consistent, BMR is positively correlated with sleep time, so that animals with a high BMR sleep for longer.
- Brain mass is positively correlated with the amount of REM sleep. Closely linked to this is the finding that the amount of REM sleep is positively correlated with an animal's EQ; animals with more advanced brains in evolutionary terms have more REM sleep.
- Animals who sleep in more dangerous places have less sleep overall and in particular less REM sleep.
- Herbivores have less REM sleep and less TST than carnivores.

The evolutionary/ecological approach to the functions of sleep tries to take into account an animal's ecological niche or lifestyle as well as a range of physiological characteristics. By doing this, it cannot be criticized as being 'reductionist', that is, it does not try to reduce the functions of sleep to one particular variable. It tries to account for sleep in terms of the animal in its natural habitat.

However, a downside of this approach is that it has to take so many variables into account and many of these variables clearly interact with each other. For instance, as mentioned above, herbivores can generally be seen as prey animals, but they can be large or small, while some sleep in safe locations and others in dangerous locations, and some are relatively advanced in evolutionary terms and some are relatively primitive. So for any one species, we have to try and balance all these different variables.

Studying scientifically

Interestingly, one of the animals often quoted to be a problem for any of the ecological accounts is the three-toed sloth. This is a relatively large mammal with a relatively low BMR, characteristics that would predict that it would not sleep more than a few hours in 24. However, some studies suggest that it can sleep for up to 20 hours a day, a problem for standard ecological accounts. A crucial point is that many of these studies were carried out on sloths kept in zoos, an artificial and usually unstimulating environment. Recent research studying sloths in their natural rain forest environment (Rattenborg et al., 2008) has shown that in fact they sleep for far less time, around six hours a day. This is line with what we would predict from the correlations outlined above between TST, body size and BMR.

This shows how important it is to control for all potential variables in a scientific study. The zoo environment seems to have been a confounding variable in the earlier research, leading to misleading results.

The evolutionary/ecological approach has identified many relevant variables that we need to take into account in explaining the functions of sleep. We now turn to the second major approach, one that focuses on restoration as the major function of sleep. Evolutionary/ecological and restoration approaches are not entirely independent. We have seen that some physiological characteristics such as BMR and EQ are associated with particular patterns of sleep, and we will refer to some of these findings in our discussion of the restoration approach.

◉ Restoration theories of sleep

Most people would agree that one function of sleep is simply to prevent you feeling tired. We have all experienced lack of sleep and the commonest effect is an increasing fatigue and a desire to sleep. In fact, there is a clear and significant relationship between prior sleep deprivation and the amount of deep NREM sleep. This observation forms the basis of the sleep homeostasis model (Borbely, 2001), which in brief proposes that we need to maintain regular levels of deep NREM sleep. If, for lifestyle or other reasons, we are deprived of it, a 'pressure' for deep NREM sleep develops. Similarly, selective deprivation of REM sleep leads to **REM rebound**, as though we need to make up for REM sleep that we have lost.

The general implication of these findings is that during sleep we recover from the effects of the previous waking day. A more scientific way of putting this is that during sleep we 'restore' some physiological processes, which may involve increasing the levels of hormones or brain neurochemicals, for example, that have been used during waking behaviour. Frustratingly, this straightforward and seemingly obvious hypothesis has been difficult to prove.

One of the clearest predictions that this hypothesis leads to is that extended periods of sleep deprivation will have significant effects. This idea has been explored in a variety of different ways.

In one of the most influential studies, Rechtschaffen et al. (1983) deprived rats of sleep and found that after a few days there were few noticeable effects, but that the animals eventually died within two or three weeks. We should note that it would be very difficult to obtain ethical permission for such studies today. To deprive rats of sleep, Rechtschaffen et al. kept them on a revolving platform, set up so that whenever they fell asleep they would fall into a pool of water. This procedure is extremely stressful and it is possible that the fatal effects of sleep deprivation in this study were due to the highly stressful procedures involved.

Interestingly, although the sleep deprived rats showed a variety of physiological changes, no single cause of death could be identified. Ideas included decreases in body temperature and a weakening of the body's immune system. This last hypothesis has been supported by studies showing that sleep deprivation in rats leads to a 20% reduction in white blood cells, a key component of the immune system (Zager et al., 2007). It may be significant that sleep deprivation in humans has been shown to have a similar effect on the immune system (Irwin et al., 1996). Although the Rechtschaffen et al. study provoked a great deal of controversy and stimulated interest in the effects of deprivation, the extreme methods used and the fact that the physiology of rats differs in many ways from that of humans makes it less relevant to theories of sleep function in humans. More direct evidence comes from studies of sleep deprivation in people.

Effects of sleep deprivation in humans

In 1959, an American DJ called Peter Tripp raised money for charity by trying to stay awake for 200 hours. During this period, he was housed in a glass booth in New York, making radio broadcasts. He was also under continual observation to try to prevent him sleeping. After just a few days of sleep deprivation, he showed signs of disorientation, with slurred speech, hallucinations and paranoid delusions. Towards the end of his remarkable efforts, he believed his food was drugged and he became extremely uncooperative with the observers. He made it to 201 hours, at which time his EEG showed all the characteristics of sleep, even though he was still apparently awake. He then slept for 24 hours and woke up feeling fully restored (Dement, 1976).

A few years later, in 1964, an American student called Randy Gardner beat Tripp's record by staying awake for 264 hours. Over this period, he did show some problems with blurred vision, some memory problems and disorganized speech, and towards the end he also became mildly paranoid. At the end of these 11 days of sleep deprivation, and before sleeping, he was able to answer questions at a press conference lucidly. On his first night's sleep, Gardner slept for about 15 hours, and on the second for about 10 hours, and was then apparently fully recovered. Overall, he regained about a quarter of the sleep he had lost, but it is significant that he recovered about two-thirds of deep NREM and about half of REM sleep (Dement, 1976).

These two dramatic case studies have caught the public imagination. Scientifically, of course, they leave a lot to be desired. Although continuously observed, it is possible they may have had micro-sleeps, and ideally they should have had continuous monitoring of EEG and other physiological measures. However, we can draw some tentative conclusions on the effects of total sleep deprivation (TSD):

- After long periods of TSD, people can recover quickly, with no apparent long-term effects
- During TSD, there are clear effects on psychological functioning, but these effects vary greatly between individuals
- Although there is sleep recovery after TSD, only a small proportion of the sleep lost is actually recovered. This recovery includes higher proportions of REM and the deep stages of NREM than the light stages of NREM.

There are other case studies relevant to the effects of sleep deprivation. For instance, **fatal familial insomnia** (FFI) is a rare condition running in families. The person has normal sleep patterns until middle age and then develops almost complete insomnia (failure to sleep). The condition is fatal, with the person dying within a few years of the onset of the insomnia. Although the precise cause is unknown, the condition does involve damage to the thalamus of the brain. This condition seems to have some parallels with Rechtschaffen et al.'s sleep deprived rats, in that in both instances, TSD results in death. But the fatal effects of TSD in the rats cannot be separated from the stress of the experimental method, and in FFI we cannot link the fatal outcome to sleep deprivation rather than to brain damage. It is difficult to establish the precise causes of death in FFI as cases are so rare.

Less dramatic, but more important from the scientific point of view are carefully controlled laboratory studies of sleep deprivation in humans. Such studies involve the sleep laboratory and polysomnography, described at the start of this chapter. Volunteer participants stay in the laboratory with constant EEG monitoring to check their state of brain arousal. In many of the studies, they are required to perform cognitive tasks involving vigilance, memory and attention at regular intervals. These allow us to assess the effects of sleep deprivation on cognitive functions under controlled conditions.

Jim Horne (1988), British sleep researcher, has reviewed over 50 such studies and drawn a number of important conclusions:

- Human participants show few if any impairments after deprivation for two or three days on cognitive tasks; such a task would be one in which they have to detect a shorter tone in a series of longer tones (Horne and Pettitt, 1985). They do have to be more motivated than non-deprived participants, for instance in the Horne and Pettitt study, they were given financial incentives to maintain performance. After longer periods of deprivation though, effects on memory and attention cannot be avoided.
- There appear to be few if any effects of moderate sleep deprivation on the body's physiological processes. The effects of deprivation appear to concentrate on brain function.
- After sleep deprivation, participants recover more REM and the deeper stages of NREM sleep than the lighter stages of NREM.

Oswald's restoration theory

Ian Oswald is another important British sleep researcher; he proposed one of the first systematic restoration theories of the function of sleep. He based this theory (Oswald, 1969, 1980) on the observation that people who had suffered damage to the brain, for example through a drug over-dose, spent more time in REM sleep as they recovered. He also noted that during deep NREM sleep, there was a large increase in the release of the growth hormone from the pituitary gland. This hormone has a range of actions on the body, but is particularly concerned with maintaining physiological systems. From these and other observations, Oswald concluded that deep NREM sleep was a time for restoration of bodily tissues. The fact that REM sleep is increased in patients recovering from brain damage led him to conclude that REM sleep was a time for restoration of the brain. So Oswald's theory proposes that REM and deep NREM have evolved for different purposes; during REM, brain circuits are restored, and during deep NREM bodily tissues are restored.

As we saw above, the findings from studies of sleep deprivation, and in particular Horne's (1988) review, were that sleep deprivation affected brain function (as demonstrated in various cognitive tasks), but there was little evidence for any effects on the body's physiological systems. It is also worth emphasizing that the case studies of Peter Tripp and Randy Gardner again demonstrated that prolonged sleep deprivation affected brain functioning but not the body's physiological functions. They both experienced symptoms such as hallucinations, incoherence and confusion, symptoms reflecting abnormalities of brain processing. More recent reviews have confirmed that sleep deprivation has clear effects on cognitive functions such as attention and working memory, but there are significant individual differences in vulnerability to these effects (Durmer and Dinges, 2005).

Based on these findings, Horne (1988) concluded that sleep was essentially a time for restoration and maintenance of the brain. He also pointed out that recovery after total sleep deprivation was concentrated on REM and the deeper slow wave stages of NREM. He therefore proposed that these two phases of sleep, REM and deep NREM, represented what he called **core sleep**, while he referred to the lighter stages of NREM as **optional sleep**. Core sleep is essential for the restoration of brain processes; optional sleep, as its name implies, is not essential for normal functioning of either the brain or the body. It may play a role in ensuring that the animal remains quiet and inconspicuous, along the lines of Meddis's protection from danger hypothesis. The two restoration theories of Oswald and Horne are obviously closely related, as shown in Table 3.1.

The key difference between these two theories is Oswald's suggestion that deep NREM is essential for restoration of the body's physiological processes. A straightforward prediction from this hypothesis is that the more bodily resources used up during the day, the more deep NREM sleep you should have during the night. In a study of marathon runners, Shapiro et al. (1981) found that they did sleep longer and spent more time in deep NREM after running a marathon, a finding that clearly supports Oswald's theory. Other studies, though, have found that the effects of physical exercise are that people go to sleep faster, but do not sleep any longer than normal.

Horne	Oswald
■ Sleep deprivation affects brain function but doesn't obviously affect the body's physiological systems	■ People who suffer damage to the brain spend more time in REM sleep during recovery
■ Sleep is essentially a time for restoration and maintenance of the brain	■ During deep NREM sleep, a large increase in the release of the growth hormone from the pituitary gland can be observed
■ Recovery after total sleep deprivation is focused on REM and the deeper stages of NREM sleep	■ Deep NREM sleep is therefore linked to the restoration of bodily tissues
■ REM and deep NREM are therefore 'core' sleep, lighter stages of NREM are 'optional' sleep	■ REM sleep is linked to the restoration of the brain
■ Core sleep is essential for the maintenance of brain processes	

Table 3.1 Comparing Oswald and Horne's restoration theories of sleep

The surge of growth hormone release during deep NREM also seems to support Oswald's view. However, it has been pointed out that the growth hormone does not work alone in maintaining bodily tissues. Proteins are the building blocks of virtually all cells and tissues in the body. Proteins are part of our diet, however, they are only available for use in the body for a few hours after a meal; after that they are absorbed into bodily tissues. As our last meal of the day is usually three to four hours before we go to sleep, the available protein levels during sleep would be very low and little would be available for the growth hormone to work with. This does not support the idea that body restoration is a crucial function of deep NREM.

There is clear agreement between Oswald and Horne on the role of REM in the maintenance and restoration of brain function. We have already seen the evidence from the studies of sleep deprivation, as sleep deprivation preferentially affects brain processes, while sleep recovery particularly involves REM. It is also supported by studies that deprive participants specifically of REM sleep (by waking them up whenever the EEG indicates that they are entering a phase of REM). When allowed to sleep, such participants show REM rebound, an overall increase in the amount of REM, indicating the importance of REM sleep. An involvement of REM in brain maintenance can also account for one of the most striking observations on the characteristics of sleep.

Although we consider life span changes in sleep later, we need to refer at this stage to the neonate (newborn baby). At birth, babies will sleep for between 16 and 20 hours a day and 50% of this sleep will be REM. In adults, the proportion of REM sleep is about 25%. So, an obvious question is why does the baby need this high proportion of REM sleep? The most popular explanations revolve around two obvious characteristics of the newborn baby:

1   Its brain is growing at an alarming rate. New neurons, and in particular new synaptic connections between neurons, are multiplying rapidly. This expansion of the brain's networks clearly requires large amounts of the building blocks of brain tissue, that is, proteins, and the expenditure of large amounts of energy.
2   The baby is taking in and processing huge amounts of information from the environment. Cognitive development during the first year is incredibly rapid.

It seems likely therefore that the higher proportion of REM in infants is closely linked either to the physiological demands of brain growth and/or the processing demands of cognitive development. In fact, these two possibilities are hard to disentangle as the growth in brain networks goes hand in hand with the increases in information processing, and one depends upon the other. The fact that the proportion of REM decreases as the brain physically matures suggests that it might be more related to the physiological processes of brain growth rather than to information processing.

An argument that has been used against the hypothesis that REM sleep is involved in brain growth and restoration is that energy consumption in the brain during REM sleep is about the same as it is in the waking state. But this argument ignores the fact that restoration may well involve the manufacture of fresh brain neurochemicals and perhaps the growth of new synaptic connections. These processes inevitably involve energy expenditure. The point perhaps becomes clearer if we compare REM and NREM sleep. We have seen that energy conservation has been a popular explanation for sleep, especially in small animals with high metabolic rates. Energy expenditure in REM is high, but energy expenditure and arousal decrease significantly in NREM, especially the deeper, slow wave stages. Total energy conservation in sleep has been estimated to be around 15% (Lesku et al., 2008), not a dramatic amount but significant. So energy conservation may be an important function of sleep, but it does not contradict the hypothesis that the specific function of REM sleep is related to the maintenance of brain networks. It is clear that given two such different phases of sleep, it would be simplistic to look for a single function of sleep.

Evolutionary/ecological and restoration approaches

It is important to realize that evolutionary/ecological and restoration approaches to the functions of sleep are not necessarily alternatives. Since the widespread use of the sleep laboratory, research into restoration hypotheses has focused on human participants and the relative roles of REM and NREM sleep. The evolutionary/ecological approach, in contrast, has investigated a wide range of different species and looked at a range of ecological variables such as trophic position and sleep site. There are, of course, overlapping areas; we have already seen that there is a positive correlation between REM sleep and brain expansion, suggesting a link between REM sleep and high-level cognitive processes. This matches Horne's idea of REM sleep being particularly important for brain function.

Sleep studies using humans largely ignore the sorts of variables important in the ecological approach. This is predictable as humans in general are neither predator nor prey, and most of them sleep in safe locations. This is not to say that the sleep patterns of modern humans have not been affected by our evolutionary heritage. Early in our evolutionary history, humans would have lived in dangerous environments and their sleeping patterns would have reflected this. Energy conservation also would have been an important function throughout their evolutionary history.

So there is no simple answer to the functions of sleep. In humans, sleep patterns are a result of our relatively large body size, moderate metabolic rate and high degree of encephalization. It also seems that REM sleep may have particularly important functions in relation to brain growth and restoration.

◉ Sleep and learning

Another popular idea in relation to sleep is that it somehow improves learning. The extreme of this view is that you can actually learn while you are sleeping – having an account of developmental psychology droning on your iPod through the night means that you wake up with a perfect memory of Bowlby and Rutter's work on attachment theory. There is no evidence that this can happen.

However, we have seen that hypotheses of the functions of sleep often refer to brain restoration, neurotransmitters and new synapses. This is particularly linked to REM sleep. When we learn, it is certain that the physiological bases of new learning involve neurotransmitters and the formation and strengthening of synaptic connections. So there has been a persistent interest in the possible links between sleep, memory and learning.

One problem with early research in this area was controlling for possible confounding factors. Contemporary research makes use of the carefully controlled environment of the sleep laboratory. This enables participant's sleep patterns to be carefully monitored, and they can also be selectively deprived of, for instance, REM sleep. For instance, Karni et al. (1994) used a simple task in which participants had to discriminate between simple line patterns. They then let the participants sleep, and used selective deprivation of REM and deep NREM – waking participants up when they entered a phase of one or the other – to show that memory for the task was affected by the loss of REM sleep, but not by deprivation of NREM sleep. This would suggest that memory consolidation is dependent on the occurrence of REM sleep.

Using a slightly more complicated motor task in which participants had to learn sequences of keyboard key presses, Walker et al. (2002) supported a role for sleep in learning and memory by showing that memory for the task improved after a period of sleep, but not after an equal period of wakefulness. Memory improvement was positively correlated with the amount of stage 2 NREM.

There is clear evidence for a role for sleep in memory and learning. Unfortunately, evidence up to now has come from simple perceptual or motor tasks. Studies using more complicated forms of learning, for example learning word lists, or problem-solving tasks, have produced inconsistent results (Walker and Stickgold, 2004).

Sleep across the life span

Changes in the amount and characteristics of sleep across the human life span may indirectly tell us something about the functions of sleep. We have already seen how the high proportion of REM sleep in babies needs to be explained by a satisfactory theory.

Sleep is a circadian rhythm and in adults the normal sleep pattern is synchronized with the light–dark cycle through its sensitivity to the exogenous zeitgeber of light. Newborn babies are not born with their biological rhythm synchronized in this way, so the first year of life is a time of major changes in the amount and patterning of sleep. By the end of the first year, the adult circadian pattern of sleep and waking is beginning to appear. The baby is sleeping for around six to eight hours at night, although there may still be daytime naps of one or two hours. The proportion of REM sleep has reduced from around 50% at birth to around the adult proportion of about 25%. By the age of two, the adult circadian pattern and proportion of REM sleep become fully established.

Changes in sleep patterns during the first two years are the most significant of any across the life span. There is substantial research evidence for further changes, although a major problem is that individuals differ greatly in the amount and patterning of sleep at particular ages and also in how they change over the years. So one has to be cautious in generalizing from any single study.

Ohayon et al. (2004) combined the results of 65 different studies and identified a number of general trends in sleep patterns between the ages of 5 and 102:

- There was a highly significant decrease in the percentage of deep NREM from 24% of total sleep time (TST) at age 5 to 9% at age 70.
- The proportion of REM sleep fell gradually over the life span from 25% of TST at age 5 to 19% at age 70. Other studies have supported this observation (Floyd et al., 2007).
- The proportions of the lighter stages of NREM (stages 1 and 2) showed slight but steady increases over the lifetime. Stage 1 increased from 5.8% at age 5 to 6.8% at age 70. Stage 2 REM increased from 47% at age 5 to 55% at age 70.
- Over the lifetime, TST decreases steadily, with the average TST for a 5-year-old being 470 minutes, and for a 70-year-old, the average TST being 370 minutes.

Other studies have investigated sleep in particular age groups. Recently, for instance, there has been a great deal of interest in sleep in adolescents. The adolescent years are a time when there is a surge in brain development, in particular the growth of new connections. If sleep (especially REM) is necessary for brain growth and maintenance, as discussed previously, then it could be argued that the stage of adolescence would require relatively more sleep.

However, adolescence is also a time of major psychological and social changes, some of which can severely affect sleep patterns. These include increases in school work, membership of school teams and social activities. Over the past decade, TV and computer use for social networking are seen as major factors in disrupting adolescent sleeping habits (Crowley et al., 2007). This study found that the typical adolescent slept less during the week but made up for it by sleeping longer at weekends. Previous studies have also found that adolescents slept on average less than other adults (Wolfson and Carskadon, 1998). The combination of disrupting biological rhythms by sleeping less during the week and more at weekends, together with an overall reduction in sleep time, would be particularly significant during a time of rapid brain growth. It has been suggested that the school day should start later to allow adolescents to catch up with their sleep loss; although this sounds rather silly, it does have a certain logic behind it.

There has also been interest in the changes in sleep patterns associated with old age. It has been firmly established that, apart from the changes noted in Ohayon et al.'s study, a common problem is a decrease in **sleep efficiency**, which is the ratio of time spent actually asleep compared with the time actually in bed. Low sleep efficiency implies that although you may be in bed for a full eight hours, you may only be getting four or five hours sleep. In old age, this is mainly due to repeated periods of waking during the night (Vitiello, 2006). Disturbed sleep at night-time leads to feelings of tiredness and fatigue and increased frequency of napping during the day.

It has been proposed that the increased frequency of night-time waking in old age may not be a natural deterioration of sleep control systems. It often seems to be associated with illness or the medications taken to treat illness. Studies on healthy older people find that night-time waking is rare (Ancoli-Israel et al., 2008). If this is true, frequent night-time waking in old age would probably qualify as a secondary insomnia (see Chapter 4).

Summary

- Sleep research was revolutionized by the introduction of the sleep laboratory and polysomnography.
- Classic work by Dement, Kleitman and Aserinsky in the 1950s identified the different phases of sleep and the association between REM sleep and dreaming.
- Sleep control mechanisms in the brainstem include the ascending reticular activating system, the locus coeruleus and the raphe nuclei. Neurotransmitters involved include noradrenaline and serotonin.
- The suprachiasmatic nucleus and the pineal gland coordinate the links between the sleep–waking cycle and the zeitgeber daylight.
- General evolutionary / ecological accounts include Meddis's safety from predation and Webb's hibernation model.
- Detailed reviews show that amount of REM sleep is related to brain mass, total sleep time is related to basal metabolic rate, while carnivores have more REM and more sleep overall than herbivores.
- Oswald and Horne both propose restoration accounts of sleep. Oswald suggests that REM sleep is for brain restoration and deep NREM sleep for body restoration. Horne concludes that REM sleep is for brain restoration, while body restoration takes place during relaxed wakefulness. Sleep deprivation studies support a role for REM sleep in brain restoration.
- There is some evidence for a role for sleep in learning and memory consolidation, but studies have used only simple learning tasks.
- There is a variety of sleep patterns across the animal kingdom. Explanations are likely to involve both ecological and restoration factors.
- Across the life span, there is a gradual reduction in the amounts of stage 3 and 4 deep NREM and REM, and also in total sleep time. There is some increase in stages 1 and 2 NREM.

Chapter 4

Disorders of sleep

👁 Introduction

Do you find yourself yawning during the day, or dozing off while watching TV? Do you feel irritable and sleepy during the day? Do people say you look tired? Are your reactions slow? Do you feel like taking a nap during the day? Do you drink a lot of caffeine to stay alert? Do you hit the snooze button on your alarm to buy yourself just a few more moments in bed? Do you find it difficult to get to sleep?

If the answer to any of these questions was yes, this suggests you are lacking in sleep. Everyone suffers from loss of sleep from time to time, but while short-term loss of sleep can be corrected by getting more sleep to overcome the deficit, problems with sleep that occur on a regular basis can indicate the presence of a sleep disorder that requires medical or psychological treatment. Given the pressures of modern life, such as work and family responsibilities and increased opportunities for socializing and networking, sleep disorders have become more frequent, and research into their causes and treatments has expanded accordingly.

In this chapter, we will cover:
- Classifying sleep disorders
- Insomnia
- Primary insomnia
- Secondary insomnia
- Factors influencing insomnia
- Hypersomnia
- Narcolepsy
- Sleepwalking

👁 Classifying sleep disorders

The twentieth century saw a dramatic increase in our understanding of both sleep and sleep disorders. Broadly, sleep disorders are a group of syndromes characterized by disturbances in the amount of sleep, the quality of sleep and the timing of sleep, or in behaviours or the physiological states associated with sleep.

In 2005, the American Academy of Sleep Medicine (2005) produced the *International Classification of Sleep Disorders* (ICSD-2), recognized as the main diagnostic tool by both researchers and clinicians. The ICSD-2 identifies over 70 different sleep disorders, broadly grouped into two subcategories – dyssomnias and parasomnias.

Dyssomnias

Dyssomnias are a group of disorders in which sufferers have problems with the amount, quality and timing of sleep. These problems result in people feeling tired during the day, and affect their ability to perform daily activities. Common dyssomnias include:

- **Insomnia**, in which patients experience chronic difficulties in falling asleep or in maintaining sleep
- **Hypersomnia**, which is characterized by excessive daytime sleepiness and often results in people falling asleep at inappropriate times during the day
- **Narcolepsy**, in which excessive daytime sleepiness is experienced alongside other symptoms, such as sudden, unavoidable collapse
- **Sleep apnoea**, a breathing-related sleep disorder
- **Restless legs syndrome**, in which people experience an irresistible urge to move their legs, which interrupts their sleep, and nocturnal myoclonus, cramps or twitches in the legs
- **Circadian rhythm sleep disorders**, caused by delayed or advanced sleep phases, for example shiftwork and jet lag, discussed in Chapter 2.

Parasomnias

Parasomnias are a range of disorders in which abnormal behaviours or physiological events occur either during sleep or during the transition between sleep and wakefulness. In contrast to dyssomnias, parasomnias rarely leave patients feeling sleepy the next day. Common parasomnias include:

- Sleepwalking (or **somnambulism**), in which the sleeper engages in activities that are normally associated with wakefulness, such as eating, walking around, getting dressed. They do these without being consciously aware they are performing the behaviours
- **REM sleep behavioural disorder** (RSBD), in which the sleeper acts out dreams during sleep, sometimes resulting in injury to themselves or those nearby
- Sleep talking, in which sleepers produce random speech during sleep
- Sleep terrors, in which the sleeper abruptly awakens from sleep in a state of terror
- Bruxism, in which sleepers grind their teeth involuntarily.

👁 Insomnia

Insomnia is a disorder classified by the ICSD-2 (American Academy of Sleep Medicine, 2005) as one of the dyssomnias. It is the most commonly experienced of all the sleep disorders. Estimates suggest that up to 58% of the population experience occasional episodes of insomnia , and that for around 10% of the population, the condition is chronic (long-lasting) (Ancoli-Israel and Roth, 1999; Morin and Mimeault, 1999). Although regarded by some as a rather trivial problem, the consequences of insomnia can be severe. Lack of sleep not only leaves the sufferer feeling tired, it can affect their mood, their ability to concentrate, their speed of reactions, and their ability to function normally in society.

There is no single pattern of sleep disturbance in insomnia, rather insomnia covers three different patterns of sleep disturbance. These are:

- *onset insomnia:* an inability to fall asleep at bedtime
- *middle insomnia:* an inability to maintain sleep throughout the night, together with problems returning to sleep once awake
- *terminal or late insomnia:* waking too early in the morning and being unable to return to sleep.

Regardless of the type of insomnia, the outcome is that the insomniac is left feeling tired during the day.

As well as the precise pattern of disturbance varying in insomnia, the duration of the disturbances can also differ. There are three categories:

- *transient insomnia:* where disrupted sleep is experienced for only a few days

- *short-term or acute insomnia:* when the inability to sleep normally continues for a period of between three weeks and six months
- *chronic insomnia:* where problems with sleep are long-lasting.

Diagnosis

Because so many people experience insomnia at some point in their lives, it is important to have a set of clearly defined criteria that separate those with a clinical disorder from those whose sleep problems are less serious. For insomnia to be diagnosed, at least one of the following symptoms is necessary:

- Sleep onset latency (time taken to fall asleep) is more than 30 minutes
- Sleep efficiency (the time spent asleep as a proportion of the time in bed) is less than 85% of the person's normal sleep efficiency
- An increase in the number of times the person wakes during the night.

For short-term or chronic insomnia, these symptoms should have been experienced three or more times a week, for a period of at least one month.

Although a doctor will use these criteria as a guide, insomnia is diagnosed in large part by the patient's assessment of whether the sleep they have is refreshing, and whether the resulting daytime fatigue causes emotional distress and/or impairs work, social or personal functioning.

Psychology as science → **Polysomnography**

The problem that doctors face in diagnosing insomnia is that much depends on the patient's subjective assessment of their problem. Unfortunately, people are often inaccurate in the estimates of the length of time they spend asleep, and they can find it difficult to find the words to describe their symptoms. To gain a more objective view, doctors may refer patients to a sleep laboratory for additional testing. This was described in Chapter 3, but it is worth reminding ourselves of this approach.

A sleep laboratory usually consists of several individual rooms, which can be observed from a central control area. Each is equipped with the comforts necessary for a good night's sleep and provides a quiet, dark environment that is free from disruptions. During the night, the sleep behaviour of the patient is observed and recordings of the patient's physiological state are taken. These usually include brain wave activity (the EEG, see Chapter 1), muscle movements, eye movements and heart rate. Measurement of this range of sleep variables is referred to as 'polysomnography', and the objective information gained from sleep laboratories provides the doctor with the information needed to diagnose sleep disorders correctly.

When considering the causes of insomnia, an important distinction can be made between two categories of this disorder:

1   *Primary insomnia*, in which the sleep disturbance occurs in the absence of any known medical or psychological condition that could account for the symptoms experienced. So, poor sleep is the primary problem.
2   *Secondary insomnia*, in which the sleep disturbance can be explained by a pre-existing medical or psychological condition. In other words, the insomnia is a side effect of, or secondary to, another problem.

This distinction is important not only in terms of understanding the causes of insomnia, but also has implications for treatment. If the insomnia is secondary to another disorder, it is important to treat the other disorder and not simply the insomnia.

◉ Primary insomnia

A diagnosis of primary insomnia is given only after a doctor has undertaken a detailed assessment of the patient's life history. Psychological and physical health checks allow a check on whether sleep problems are secondary to some other cause.

There are a number of different subtypes that fall within the classification of primary insomnia, each with a different underlying cause:

- *Psychophysiological insomnia:* a form of anxiety-induced insomnia, sometimes called learned or behavioural insomnia. This develops when a period of stress is accompanied by poor sleep. Together, these result in two maladaptive patterns of behaviour being learned:
  - A vicious cycle of 'trying hard to get to sleep' is established. The harder the person tries to sleep, the tenser they become, and the tenser they become, the less likely it is they will sleep
  - Bedtime habits and routines become associated (through classical conditioning) with feelings of frustration and arousal. As the

person has a history of insomnia, they anticipate the problems they will have, leading to anticipated anxiety and arousal, and so the problem persists.

Typically the problem would take this form – a person who sleeps badly at night may worry that they won't be able to function well the next day, which results in them trying even harder to sleep at night. Unfortunately, the efforts they make to sleep actually cause them to become more aroused and alert and trigger further anxious thoughts, which means sleep is even less likely.

Sometimes the learned association between bedtime habits and arousal can be quite specific, and sufferers find that they are able to sleep in novel locations, such as hotel bedrooms, where they unable to sleep in their own beds. This is because the learned associations are not present in this new sleeping environment.

- *Idiopathic insomnia:* usually begins in childhood and is a lifelong condition. It is suggested that this form of insomnia is caused by neurochemical problems in the regions of the brain that control the sleep–waking cycle (Chapter 3). This results in brain arousal patterns being dislocated from light and dark, that is, with waking patterns at night-time that prevent normal sleep.

- *Sleep state misperception:* the patient's sleep is adequate, but their perception of the time they have slept is distorted. This disparity can be identified in sleep laboratories where there is a difference between the patient's subjective assessment of their sleep time and the objective measurements. Dement and Vaughn (1999) described one patient who complained of severe insomnia and so was asked to sleep for 10 consecutive nights in a sleep laboratory. Each morning he estimated how long he had taken to fall asleep the previous night. These estimates ranged from one to four hours, with a mean of 90 minutes. However, the laboratory recordings showed that he never took more than 30 minutes to fall asleep and the mean time was only 15 minutes.

Causal factors

From the brief descriptions of these three different types, it is clear that there is no single explanation for primary insomnia. Rather, a number of causal factors are involved.

Arousal

However caused, high levels of arousal mean that it will be difficult for an individual to sleep. Although not all forms of primary insomnia are related to arousal, arousal plays a role in both idiopathic and psycho-physiological insomnia. In idiopathic insomnia, a malfunction in the brain results in arousal levels being too high for sleep to occur normally. In psychophysiological insomnia, arousal, in the form of stress, sets the scene for the maladaptive sleep-related behaviours to be learned, and from then on, ongoing anxiety maintains the disorder.

Support for the role of arousal as a causal factor in primary insomnia comes from sleep studies using polysomnography. These show that people with primary insomnia often have elevated night-time levels of cortisol (a stress hormone) and adrenocorticotropic hormone (this stimulates the secretion of cortisol). This would indicate high levels of stress-related arousal. Support also comes from studies using positron emission tomography (PET) brain scans, which indicate that people with insomnia generally have higher arousal levels both when awake and asleep (Bonnet and Arand, 1995). The role of arousal as a cause of primary insomnia is further supported by the effectiveness of treatments such as cognitive behavioural therapy (CBT) and relaxation techniques. CBT addresses anxiety-related arousal, and relaxation targets arousal levels more generally.

Learned associations

Psychophysiological insomnia suggests that primary insomnia may be a learned response. The role of learning as a cause of primary insomnia is supported by the success of stimulus control therapy as a treatment. The objective of stimulus control therapy is for the patient to learn new associations between sleep and bedtime cues, which then replace the maladjusted patterns they have learned during a time of stress. This behavioural therapy involves controlling both the sleep environment and restricting sleep, to ensure that attempts to sleep are only made when the patient is really tired.

Abnormalities of the sleep circuit in the brain

Idiopathic insomnia seems to be clearly related to a malfunction in the complex sleep control system in the brain, suggesting that such malfunctions can be a cause of primary insomnia. This view is supported by research which shows that patients with damage to areas of the brain involved in the sleep–waking cycle often suffer from insomnia (Lavie, 1996). Although drugs could, in theory, be used to address the neurochemical dysfunction in the sleep–waking circuits, the drugs currently available are not sufficiently sophisticated to target specific regions of the circuit. So, although the sleeping pills that are currently available can help when insomnia is secondary to anxiety or depression, they are not helpful in the treatment of primary insomnia.

Faulty cognition

Sleep state misperception suggests that cognitive processes play a role in the development of primary insomnia. This view is supported by the success of CBT treatments. The 'cognitive' component of cognitive behavioural therapy targets the patient's faulty perceptions of their sleep patterns. By giving the patient a more realistic picture of how they are actually sleeping, anxiety and arousal are reduced.

Genes

There is evidence that at least some forms of primary insomnia may have a genetic basis. Idiopathic insomnia, for instance, has been found to run in families (American Academy of Sleep Medicine, 2005), and a study that compared the incidence of insomnia in the families of 256 primary insomniacs reported that 72.7% of the primary insomniacs had a family history of insomnia. This compares with 24.1% of the non-insomnia group (Dauvilliers et al., 2005). This supports the idea that slight malfunctions in sleep–waking circuits can be inherited.

◉ Secondary insomnia

Secondary insomnia has been found to be a consequence of a wide range of factors, including:

- *Medical conditions* such as heart disease, high blood pressure, Wilson's syndrome, Parkinson's disease, hyperthyroidism, epilepsy and asthma have all been associated with chronic sleep problems. The particular sleep problems shown may relate either to the condition itself, or may be related to the pain and discomfort patients experience as a result of these conditions. Pain can prevent patients from finding a comfortable position to fall asleep in, and may wake them during the night when they change their sleeping position. Secondary insomnia may also result from the medication used to treat these conditions.

- *Neurological conditions* that affect patients at night can cause secondary insomnia. Nocturnal myoclonus and restless legs syndrome (RLS) can both be a cause of insomnia. Patients with nocturnal myoclonus wake up because of cramps or twitches in the legs, and RLS patients wake because they have crawly or aching feelings in their lower legs. They feel compelled to relieve these aches by moving or rubbing the leg, and often find it difficult to go back to sleep until the morning when the condition is not so severe. Both nocturnal myoclonus and RLS leave patients feeling sleepy the next day.
- *Psychological and psychiatric conditions* such as depression, anxiety, post-traumatic stress disorder, obsessive compulsive disorder and schizophrenia are frequently associated with periods of insomnia. The manic phase in patients with bipolar disorder has also been associated with sleeplessness. In fact, it has been estimated that about 40% of all those diagnosed with insomnia have a co-occurring psychological disorder (Morin and Mimeault, 1999).
- The use of *stimulant substances* that produce physiological arousal, such as psychoactive drugs, caffeine and tobacco, can cause insomnia.
- *Sleep apnoea* and *parasomnias* can disrupt sleep. For instance, those who sleepwalk or grind their teeth at night (bruxism) experience disrupted sleep.
- *Fatal familial insomnia* (FFI) is a rare genetic, neurodegenerative disease that causes an insomnia which gradually progresses from a mild disorder to a state of complete sleeplessness. It is untreatable and ultimately leads to death. This is sometimes used as evidence for the 'essential' nature of sleep (see Chapter 3). However, it is likely that death is related to the underlying neurodegenerative condition as well as to sleep loss.

◉ Factors influencing insomnia

Insomnia is a highly prevalent sleep disorder that affects the psychological wellbeing and quality of life of its sufferers. As we have already seen, many factors play a part in insomnia, and it can be helpful to consider these in terms of the specific roles they play:

- *Predisposing factors* are the inbuilt characteristics of a person that make them vulnerable to insomnia

- *Precipitating factors* are events that trigger insomnia
- *Perpetuating factors* are behaviours that help to maintain sleeplessness once it has begun.

Each of these areas are now discussed in more detail.

Predisposing factors

While precipitating factors have received much research attention, the role of predisposing factors has not received the same level of attention. A picture is, however, beginning to emerge that suggests there are a number of factors that increase people's vulnerability to insomnia.

Genes

There is evidence that some forms of insomnia have a significant genetic component. This can be seen in family studies (for example Dauvilliers et al., 2005) and twin studies. One study examined 1,042 pairs of monozygotic twins and 828 pairs of dyzygotic twins, and concluded that the heritability of insomnia was 57% (Watson et al., 2006).

The specific gene involved in insomnia has not yet been identified in humans. However, research into a type of fruit fly that sleeps for only one or two hours per day, compared to the usual 12 hours for other types of fruit fly, has identified a gene, which the researchers named 'sleepless'. This may well have implications for the understanding of insomnia in humans (Wu et al., 2008).

Personality

Personality traits may also act as a predisposing factor for secondary insomnia. Although it seems that personality traits are not directly related to the duration of sleep (Van Dongen et al., 2005; Soehner et al., 2007), research has shown that insomniacs display more signs of neuroticism (a personality trait that is significantly correlated with anxiety), internalization (meaning they internalize their concerns rather than acting them out, increasing emotional arousal and anxiety) and traits associated with perfectionism, compared with those without sleep problems (for example Kales et al., 1976; Heath et al., 1998; Van de Laar, 2010). Each of these personality factors may play a different role in different subtypes of insomnia.

Understanding the role of personality traits can be important when considering treatment options. For example, insomniacs who score highly on scales measuring mania show less improvement when undertaking psychological treatments than those whose mania scores are low. However, the specific role of personality traits in insomnia is still unclear. Although neuroticism, internalization and perfectionism may play a causal role in the development of insomnia, they could also be consequences of the disorder. To answer the question of whether they are a cause or an effect, longitudinal studies would need to be conducted. Future research is also needed to examine whether specific personality traits are associated with specific subcategories of insomnia.

Psychology as science → **Reliability and validity of personality questionnaires**

All research that investigates personality traits makes use of questionnaires. Before conducting research, the validity and reliability of these measures needs to be assessed. Validity can be established in a number of ways; for example by simply looking at the questionnaire to see if it looks as if it measures the personality dimensions it sets out to measure (face validity). Reliability is particularly important in personality tests as personality traits are stable over time, so tests taken at different times should produce similar results (test–retest reliability). In the assessment of personality questionnaires, it is also important to conduct a split-half test, in which the scores from half of the questions are correlated with the scores from the other half of the questions. If the two sets are measuring the same aspect of personality, they should correlate highly.

Chronotype

Chronotype refers to whether a person is a 'morning type' or 'evening type'. Morning types, or 'larks', have body clocks that wake them about two hours earlier and indicate it is time for sleep about two hours earlier than most. Evening types, or 'owls', generally wake two hours later and go to bed two hours later than the majority of the population. While the sleep patterns of morning and evening types are usually stable, there is some suggestion that chronotype can predispose people to insomnia. Chung et al. (2009) studied nurses who worked shifts and found the strongest predictor of sleep quality was the chronotype and not the shift schedule.

Age

Ageing increases the likelihood of insomnia (see Chapter 3 for a review of changes in sleep patterns with age). It is a common misperception that the amount of sleep required decreases dramatically as a person ages. However, it seems that the need for sleep remains largely intact but the ability to sleep for long periods is lost, with frequent night-time waking. Often the cause of age-related insomnia is an increase in physical problems such as arthritis, or it may be due to low levels of melatonin in the brain.

Gender

Women are more often diagnosed with insomnia than men. There are a number of reasons why this might be the case. It could simply be that women are more willing than men to visit their doctor and discuss health issues, or perhaps women generally have higher levels of neuroticism and anxiety. Sleep problems have also been linked to the hormonal fluctuations that women experience at different times in their lives. The changes in hormone levels experienced during the menstrual cycle, pregnancy and the menopause have physiological effects on the body that include effects on the brain mechanisms of sleep. As well as the hormonal change itself causing vulnerability, during times of hormonal change, women often experience cravings for sugary food and alcohol. These affect blood sugar levels and contribute to sleeping problems. During pregnancy, a woman has additional problems to cope with, particularly in terms of increasing anxiety as the birth approaches. This can cause problems with sleeping, as can the need for her to find new sleep positions to accommodate changes in her body shape and size.

Other sleep disorders, for example sleep apnoea

Suffering from another sleep disorder can predispose an individual to insomnia. Sleep apnoea, classified as a parasomnia, is a disorder in which sleep is disrupted due to breathing problems. Although mild problems with breathing, such as those associated with snoring, are not uncommon, in sleep apnoea the problem is severe. Normal breathing is paused for periods lasting anywhere from a few seconds to minutes, and these disruptions can occur up to 30 times an hour. During the time that breathing is paused, carbon dioxide builds up in the bloodstream. When this reaches a critical level, it is detected by chemoreceptors, receptors in the bloodstream specialized to detect specific chemicals. These receptors signal an alarm to the brain that wakes the sleeper as they gasp for air. Once normal oxygen levels are restored, the patient returns to sleep, and the process starts again.

There are two forms of the disorder – obstructive and central:

- In **obstructive sleep apnoea**, the cause of the problem is the loss of muscle tone in the sleeper's respiratory tract, which causes it to partially collapse. Although patients with this form of apnoea do not generally recall waking during the night or having problems breathing, they do complain of excessive sleepiness during the day.
- In **central sleep apnoea**, the normal control of breathing by the central nervous system is interrupted. Patients do recall waking and often find it difficult to return to sleep. Despite this, they do not generally experience excessive daytime sleepiness.

Other factors that may predispose people to insomnia include pre-existing psychological and psychiatric disorders, and medical and neurological conditions. These were reviewed earlier in relation to secondary insomnia.

It is clear that there are a number of factors that can predispose a person to insomnia, but the diathesis-stress model proposes that in many cases these factors are not sufficient in their own right to cause insomnia. The **diathesis-stress model** is a psychological theory that explains behaviour as both a result of biological and genetic factors ('nature'), and life experiences ('nurture'). We inherit a vulnerability to insomnia, but it needs some environmental stimulus to trigger the disorder.

Precipitating factors

Humans were designed to sleep at night when the world was quiet and dark. Today the world is very different and there are many environmental stressors that can act as triggers or precipitating factors for insomnia. People spend many hours commuting each day and work in highly demanding, stressful jobs. We can shop 24/7, and the introduction of the light bulb and the growth in technology means we can now be active all day, every day (see Chapter 2). Cities have become noisier places to live, and loud noise can trigger insomnia, particularly when the noises occur unpredictably. However, noise does not always inhibit sleep. White noise (a low, constant hiss) has been found to benefit people suffering from insomnia, possibly because it dulls other sounds in the environment (Lopez et al., 2002).

Besides environmental pressures, other factors can trigger insomnia:

- *Negative life events*, such as the death of a loved one, an increase in responsibility, financial problems or hospitalization, can result in stress and anxiety, which in turn can trigger insomnia

- *Unhealthy diets* increase the likelihood of insomnia, with sugar, caffeine and alcohol being particular culprits
- *International jet travel* and *change in work patterns* can produce abrupt changes in our sleep–waking pattern that can, in turn, provoke insomnia (see Chapter 2)
- *Drugs* and *alcohol* can cause problems in sleeping, and are common causes of insomnia
- Even *exercise* can be a problem, as the arousal caused by excessive activity can make it difficult to asleep, as many top athletes will testify.

Perpetuating factors

In addition to factors that leave people vulnerable to insomnia, or that precipitate the disorder, there are also factors that maintain the disorder. These perpetuating factors offer the key to understanding chronic insomnia:

- *Prescribed sleeping pills*: It may seem paradoxical that taking prescribed sleeping pills can result in even greater sleep problems, but this is what happens. The benefits these drugs offer are only short term. As the body becomes accustomed to the drug in the bloodstream, it develops tolerance and a higher dosage is needed to produce the same effect. This means that, over a period of time, the benefits decrease as the dosage increases. Continued use can result in physical and emotional dependency, and there are serious side effects associated with withdrawal from these drugs. These include anxiety, mood changes, loss of appetite and, most importantly, an increase in sleep problems.
- *Alcohol:* Alcohol is not only a precipitating factor for insomnia, it is also a perpetuating factor. It is a common misconception that alcohol aids sleep and many people with insomnia turn to alcohol as a means of overcoming their problem. However, although alcohol is a relaxant and its initial effect is to switch off adrenaline, causing a feeling of relaxation, after a few hours, the body starts to adjust and tries to regulate the effects. This interferes with the sequence and duration of sleep stages and leaves the user feeling tired and irritable in the morning. Consuming alcohol in the evening, even in moderate amounts, can also exacerbate problems such as sleep apnoea.

Other perpetuating factors include tension due to previous experiences of sleep difficulties, and heavy smoking.

I hope you have realized by now that research into the causes and treatment of insomnia is not straightforward. This is mainly because it is a complex area, but there are additional reasons why research progress has been slow.

Lack of a clear definition for insomnia

There is no doubt that people diagnosed with insomnia have disordered sleep, but do all insomniacs suffer from the same disorder? As we have seen, not only are there a number of different disordered patterns of sleep that can be classified as insomnia, but there are also a wide range of biological and psychological causes for insomnia. Because of this, some researchers suggest that insomnia is not a single sleep disorder. It may be that insomnia is a disorder that currently includes a number of more specific sleep disorders. It may also be that problems in falling asleep, maintaining sleep, and/or waking too early are symptoms of other disorders, and not sleep disorders per se.

So insomnia is a complex disorder that is difficult to define in any simple way. The lack of clear definition raises problems in a number of areas:

- *Diagnosis:* An accurate diagnosis of any disorder should be based on clear-cut criteria that specify exactly what the clinician should look for in order to label the person with that specific disorder. Without a clear definition for insomnia, it is not possible to provide a set of such criteria. Current criteria are extremely loose and encompass a large number of subcategories of insomnia. There is also considerable overlap in the criteria used to diagnose insomnia and the criteria for other disorders with similar symptoms. Because the criteria are not specific, clinicians are required to take into account the patient's subjective assessment of their quality of sleep and the level of associated distress. Any diagnosis that relies so heavily on subjective judgement is unlikely to be entirely reliable, which means that different clinicians may arrive at different diagnoses when presented with the same patient. This problem brings into question the validity and reliability of diagnostic classification systems such as the

DSM-IV and ICD-10. It is essential that a clearer definition of insomnia is found that both differentiates insomnia from similar disorders, and reliably identifies specific subtypes of insomnia.

- *Treatment:* A number of different treatments have been found to be effective in chronic primary insomnia; these include behavioural therapies, CBT and relaxation techniques. However, not all treatments have been found to be equally effective with all subtypes. It is therefore critical that reliable diagnostic criteria are developed that identify the various subtypes so that the most effective treatment can be prescribed.

- *Research:* All research requires a clear definition of the issue being investigated, but because insomnia lacks a clear definition, it is difficult to conduct research in any meaningful way. It is also difficult to generalize the findings from particular research studies. Findings may be applicable to one subtype of insomnia, but may not apply to all subtypes.

- *Assessing the scale of the problem:* Estimates have suggested that about 10% of the population are chronic insomniacs. However, because the disorder is poorly defined, this figure may not reflect the true scale of the problem.

The validity of current research methods

As well as aiding clinicians in their diagnosis, polysomnography provides researchers with a tool that allows them to investigate the nature and causes of insomnia (and other sleep disorders). This research takes place in a laboratory situation, albeit one with beds in it, and, as with all research carried out in laboratories, it is important to consider the validity of the data that is collected in this way. A number of studies have correlated the self-reported data from patients with the objective data produced in the sleep laboratory to see whether this data has external validity. Although discrepancies can be found (we saw earlier that one patient's estimate of their sleep latency was different to the polysomnography results), most studies have found a high positive correlation between self-report rating scales and laboratory measures. For example, a positive correlation was found between patients' self-report data and laboratory data in one sleep disorder, restless legs syndrome (Borreguero et al., 2004). So, it seems that data from the sleep laboratory has external validity, at least for some sleep disorders.

Directions for future research

There are many questions that remain to be addressed by future research:

- *Understanding the nature of the subtypes of insomnia:* Research that identified the unique behavioural and biological patterns associated with each subtype would allow diagnostic criteria to be developed that identified each subtype, which, in turn, would lead to the most effective treatment being prescribed.

- *Treatments:* Although biological dysfunctions have been identified, as yet drugs have proved to be ineffective in the treatment of chronic primary insomnias, although they are used successfully in some cases where insomnia is a secondary symptom. The problem lies in the effects of present-day hypnotics (sleeping tablets). These are currently far too general to address the highly specific dysfunctions that have been identified in the complex sleep–waking mechanisms of the brain. Research is needed to investigate the nature of these dysfunctions, and also to develop drugs that are more specific in their effects.

- *Gender differences:* Although statistics show that more women are diagnosed with insomnia than men, relatively little research has been conducted to investigate the reasons for this. At the moment, there are suggestions that sex hormones play a role in the development of insomnia (see earlier in this chapter), but it seems unlikely that this gender difference is due entirely to biological factors. It may be that psychological factors play an important role, for instance the possibility that women are more prepared to seek help when they have a problem. This requires further research.

- *Cultural differences:* Cultural differences have been found in some sleep disorders, but, as yet, there has been little consideration as to whether there are cultural differences in the prevalence of insomnia. If further research identifies cultural differences, it might suggest that psychological factors and life stressors play a more important role in insomnia than biological factors.

Hypersomnia

In contrast to insomnia, in which people have trouble falling asleep or staying asleep, hypersomnia (a dyssomnia) is a disorder in which people experience an excessive need to sleep. The primary symptoms are excessive daytime sleepiness (EDS) and prolonged periods of night-time sleep.

Hypersomniacs can sleep for up to 12 hours each night, during which they experience abnormally long periods of non-REM sleep (Chapter 3) lasting between one and two hours. They still find it difficult to wake up, and generally feel disorientated and groggy when they do. Because of this, the disorder is sometimes called 'sleep drunkenness'. Despite the long periods they spend sleeping at night, hypersomniacs also experience irresistible urges to nap during the day. The timing of these urges is unpredictable, and they often fall asleep at inconvenient moments such as when eating, driving, cooking or working. Unlike the daytime naps that non-sufferers may take to relieve the sleepiness caused by a lack of night-time sleep, these naps offer no relief from the feelings of sleepiness in hypersomniacs. In addition to disrupted sleep patterns, hypersomniacs may also experience anxiety, increased irritation, decreased energy, restlessness, slow thinking, slow speech, loss of appetite, hallucinations and memory difficulties.

Hypersomnia is an uncommon disorder, with less than 5% of adults complaining of excessive daytime sleepiness. Its onset is insidious (gradual, so you can be unaware of it at first). Symptoms typically appear before the age of 25, and it is found more commonly in men than women. Because of the nature of the disorder, many patients lose the ability to function adequately in family, social, occupational, or other settings.

Hypersomnia can take two forms, both of which have the same symptom profile but differ in the frequency with which symptoms occur:

1 *Primary hypersomnia*, in which symptoms are experienced continually for months or even years
2 *Recurrent hypersomnia*, in which periods of hypersomnia are mixed with normal sleep–waking cycles. The best-known form of recurrent hypersomnia is the rare condition, Kleine–Levin syndrome. Patients with this condition experience two to three days of sleeping for 18–20 hours a day, yet still wake up feeling tired. These extended periods of sleep are accompanied by other disturbed behaviours including hypersexuality, compulsive eating and irritability. They then return to normal patterns of sleep and behaviour until the next episode occurs.

Diagnosis

The diagnosis of hypersomnia requires the following attributes:

- Excessive sleepiness must be experienced for at least one month, or less if the disorder is recurrent, either in terms of prolonged night-time sleep and/or daytime sleep episodes that occur almost daily.

- Excessive sleepiness must cause significant distress or impairment of social, occupational, or other important areas of functioning.
- Excessive sleepiness cannot be attributed to another mental disorder (for example depression), is not due to inadequate amounts of sleep, or to another sleep disorder (for example narcolepsy or sleep apnoea), is not the direct effect of a substance (for example recreational drugs, alcohol or medication), and is not due to any general medical condition.

Causes of hypersomnia

Currently, the causes of hypersomnia are unclear, although a number of factors have been identified, all of which may contribute to the disorder at some level:

- It appears that some people may have a genetic predisposition to hypersomnia, although this is not the case for all sufferers
- Functional brain problems, such as a dysfunction of sleep–waking mechanisms.

Although, as noted above, hypersomnia secondary to other identifiable factors or conditions is not technically classified as clinical hypersomnia, it is still important to recognize the role of such factors. These include:

- Structural changes in the brain caused by tumours, head trauma, or other damage to the central nervous system
- Infection, for example influenza
- Excessive sleepiness can be a side effect of certain medications, for example psychotropic medication prescribed for depression, anxiety or bipolar disorder, or of withdrawal from some medications
- Abuse of recreational drugs or alcohol
- Medical conditions, including multiple sclerosis, depression, encephalitis, epilepsy or obesity
- Other sleep disorders, particularly narcolepsy and sleep apnoea.

Treatment

As the cause of primary clinical hypersomnia is often unknown, the available treatment options are limited. Currently, treatment consists of the use of stimulant drugs, such as amphetamines and modafinil, to increase alertness during the day. Behavioural changes may also be tried, such as limiting the number and length of daytime naps, and improved sleep hygiene, that is, trying to improve sleep habits. This might involve:

- using the bedroom only for sleep and bedroom activities such as sex, and not using it for watching TV or work
- going to bed and waking at the same, regular times, in association with reducing daytime naps.

◉ Narcolepsy

Narcolepsy is, perhaps, the most dramatic of all the sleep disorders that involve excessive daytime sleepiness (EDS). The main symptoms of narcolepsy are:

- *Excessive daytime sleepiness:* Patients experience an irresistible tendency to fall asleep, even in unlikely circumstances such as during a meal or while in conversation. These 'daytime sleep attacks' are quite brief, typically lasting between 10–20 minutes, and although the patient wakes feeling refreshed, they start to feel sleepy again very quickly (this pattern can be contrasted with hypersomnia, where daytime naps offer little relief from feelings of sleepiness).
- *Abnormal REM sleep:* Narcoleptics have unique sleep cycles in which they enter the REM phase of sleep at the beginning of sleep, even when that sleep occurs during the day. The usual ultradian sleep pattern (see Chapter 3) is for REM sleep to follow a period in the light stages of non-REM sleep.

Patients may also experience a number of other symptoms:

- **Cataplexy** (sudden loss of muscle control): Narcoleptics often experience a sudden loss of muscle control while awake, leading to physical collapse.
- *Hallucinations:* Vivid, sometimes frightening, visual or auditory sensations may be experienced either just before falling asleep (hypnogogic hallucinations) or immediately after waking up (hypnopompic hallucinations).
- *Sleep paralysis:* This is an inability to move that sometimes occurs during the transition from sleep to wakefulness.

- *Micro-sleeps:* These are very brief sleep episodes during which patients continue to function (talk, put things away and so on) and then awaken with no memory of these activities.
- *Night-time wakefulness:* People with narcolepsy may have periods of wakefulness at night, with hot flushes, elevated heart rate, and sometimes intense alertness.

Two of the most common symptoms, EDS and cataplexy, appear to be connected to emotional states, as both can be triggered by the experience of intense emotions, such as laughter, sadness, surprise, frustration or anger.

Estimates suggest that narcolepsy affects about 1 in 2,000 people. Most experience their first symptoms between the ages of 10 and 25, although about 18% of patients are less than 10 years old, and some people are more than 30 years old when they experience symptoms for the first time.

Socioeconomic impact

Narcolepsy is a disabling disorder that can have a devastating effect on the lives of its victims. It can affect physical wellbeing, as even everyday activities are potentially dangerous if you fall asleep while performing them. It affects mental health, often resulting in anxiety and depression. Cognitive abilities are compromised as patients generally experience memory problems and have difficulty in concentrating. Social and professional relationships are affected, particularly when others are unfamiliar with the condition and assume that the sufferer is lazy, rude or faking their excessive need for sleep. Intimate relationships can also suffer, particularly as extreme sleepiness can result in low sex drive and impotence. Studies have shown that even treated narcoleptic patients are often markedly impaired in the areas of work, leisure, interpersonal relations, and are more prone to accidents.

Diagnosis

When diagnosing narcolepsy, a doctor will first consider the self-reported symptoms, which should include:

- Irresistible attacks of refreshing sleep that occur daily for at least three months
- The presence of either one or both of the following: cataplexy and/ or hallucinations or sleep paralysis experienced during the transition between sleeping and waking.

In addition to considering self-reported symptoms, the doctor needs to exclude the possibility that the sleep disturbance could be secondary to substances such as drugs or alcohol, or could be a side effect of another medical or psychological condition.

Although the diagnostic criteria seem clear, narcolepsy can be a difficult disorder to identify, and it is often years before a correct diagnosis is made. One problem is that people fail to recognize EDS as a symptom of a sleep disorder and do not consult a doctor. Even when they do consult a doctor, they often only report symptoms of EDS. This may be because they have failed to recognize other symptoms as being related to EDS, or it may be because the symptoms are too mild for them to notice; either way this can lead to a misdiagnosis. It is only when a patient reports cataplexy (the sudden loss of muscle control) that it is immediately apparent that the patient is suffering from narcolepsy, as cataplexy is the unique symptom.

Because diagnosis on the basis of self-report is so problematic, doctors sometimes use two diagnostic tests to help:

1 *Nocturnal polysomnography* – an overnight test conducted in a sleep laboratory in which the electrical activity of the brain, heart and muscles are recorded.
2 *Multiple sleep latency test* – also conducted in a sleep clinic and measures how long it takes the patient to fall asleep during the day.

Together, the results of these tests indicate the length of time it takes for the patient to fall asleep at night and during the day, which, in the case of narcoleptics, would be expected to be very brief. They also indicate the positioning of the REM phase in the ultradian sleep cycle, and allow for other causes of daytime sleepiness, such as sleep apnoea, to be excluded.

Causes of narcolepsy

Although the disorder has long been recognized, it was not until the middle of the last century that explanations began to be offered to account for these extraordinary patterns of behaviour. One of the earliest explanations came from the psychodynamic perspective. This suggested that the purpose of the sudden attacks of sleepiness was to disguise sexual fantasies (Lehrman and Weiss, 1943). As with most psychodynamic explanations, this hypothesis is not easily tested; however, it did acknowledge the link between narcolepsy and dream sleep states. Then there are biological explanations, which have more validity.

REM sleep hypothesis

The earliest biological explanation for narcolepsy examined the link between the disorder and the REM stage of sleep, prompted by the observation that there are clear overlaps between the two. The visual and auditory hallucinations that patients report during the sleep–wake transition have a dreamlike quality similar to dreaming in REM sleep. The muscular paralysis is also similar to the paralysis found during REM sleep; this prevents people moving around and acting out their dreams (Chapter 3). In 1960, Vogel confirmed that narcolepsy was a REM sleep-related disorder when he found that sleep patterns in narcolepsy were disrupted. In narcolepsy, REM sleep occurs at the start of sleep, rather than after about 90 minutes and a period in the lighter stages of non-REM sleep, as in the normal sleep pattern.

Genes

More recently, scientists have made much progress in determining the specific mechanisms involved in narcolepsy. Early research was conducted using strains of genetically modified dogs, which were bred to mimic the patterns of human narcoleptics. These dogs showed behavioural symptoms similar to those found in human patients, in that the dogs would collapse following emotional excitement (such as the appearance of food) and pass directly into REM sleep (Aldrich, 1998). The fact that it was possible to breed such strains of dogs suggested that heredity may play a role in the disorder.

More recently, a candidate gene was been identified. This gene is found in an area of chromosome 6, and is known as the HLA (human leukocyte antigen) complex gene. The purpose of the HLA gene is to help coordinate our immune system. To do this, it produces molecules, found on the surface of white blood cells, which coordinate the immune response. These molecules differ slightly from individual to individual, which explains why immune systems differ slightly between individuals. In 2009, researchers at Stanford University School of Medicine identified a specific subtype of the HLA complex gene (the HLA-DQB1*0602 subtype), which appeared to be a marker for narcolepsy (Hallmayer et al., 2009). Over 90% of narcoleptics whose symptoms included cataplexy were found to carry this gene. However, not all research has supported genes as an explanation for narcolepsy.

Family and twin studies do not suggest that heredity plays a significant role in narcolepsy (Mignot, 1998). Not all narcoleptics carry the identified variant of the HLA complex gene, and the gene is quite common in people who do not suffer from narcolepsy (Mignot et al., 1997). Cross-cultural research also questions the role of genes. The reported incidence of the disorder in Japan is almost 2% of the population, while in Europe the figure is closer to 0.05%. There is no evidence for major differences in the genetic makeup of Japanese and European populations, so unless the differences in these figures can be accounted for by differences in the way the disorder is diagnosed, it suggests that the disorder cannot be the result of genes alone and environmental factors must play some role. So, although the ability to breed narcoleptic dogs suggests that the role of heredity may be important, human research suggests that other factors must be involved.

Hypocretin

Hypocretin (also known as orexin) is a neurotransmitter (chemical messenger in the brain) involved in arousal and the regulation of sleep. Only 10,000–20,000 cells in the entire human brain (out of many billions) secrete hypocretin molecules. These are located in a subregion of the hypothalamus, an area located deep in the base of the brain. The hypothalamus regulates many basic functions such as the release of hormones, blood pressure, sexual and reproductive behaviours, food intake regulation and sleep.

Animal studies, using genetically modified dogs, suggested that the symptoms of narcolepsy could be caused by the absence of hypocretin (Chemelli et al., 1999) or the absence of the receptor to which the hypocretin molecules attach (Lin et al., 1999). Human studies have also reported very low levels of hypocretin in samples of cerebrospinal fluid (CSF) from narcoleptic patients (Nishimo et al., 2000); CSF is secreted by the brain into chambers in the centre of the brain (the ventricles) that connect with the spinal canal running through the spinal cord. Samples of CSF can be extracted from the spinal canal using a technique known as a 'lumbar puncture', and tested for various chemicals. Low levels of hypocretin in CSF suggest low levels in brain tissue.

What causes low hypocretin levels? Besides possible genetic factors, low levels of hypocretin could be caused by a number of factors, including:

- infection
- diet
- contact with toxins such as pesticides

- brain injuries due to conditions such as brain tumours or strokes, although only rarely have cases been reported of narcolepsy arising as a consequence of such structural damage.

Perhaps the most promising explanation links the HLA gene subtype found in many narcoleptics and low levels of hypocretin. The HLA subtype (HLA-DQB1*0602), which was identified as being carried by the vast majority of patients, has been shown to increase the risk of an autoimmune response to neurons in the brain that produce hypocretin. An autoimmune response is when the immune system attacks the body's healthy cells rather than fighting off external infection. Examples of autoimmune disorders include multiple sclerosis and rheumatoid arthritis. Most autoimmune disorders are associated with specific HLA subtypes, for instance about 70% of the patients with multiple sclerosis have HLA-DR2.

Recent studies have shown that the hypocretin-containing cells are reduced in the brains of many narcoleptic patients. The most likely explanation for this is that they have been destroyed by an autoimmune attack (Mignot, 2001), and this interpretation is supported by the presence of the HLA-DQB*0602 subtype in many narcoleptic patients. For some reason, this HLA subtype provokes the body's immune system into attacking the hypocretin-containing cells in the hypothalamus. However, it is important to remember that many people with narcolepsy do not carry that particular HLA subtype, so this would not explain all cases of narcolepsy.

Psychology as science → **Applying research**

Research into the causes of narcolepsy has provided us with a greater understanding of this sleep disorder and has allowed sleep researchers to gain further insights into the mechanisms that control sleep, but can these findings be applied to improve diagnosis and treatment for sufferers?

Improving diagnosis

There are two possible candidates identified through research studies that may help in the diagnosis of narcolepsy:

- *HLA typing:* As we have seen, there is a specific HLA gene subtype (HLA-DQB1*0602) associated with narcolepsy, so could identifying carriers of this subtype help refine the diagnosis of this disorder? Unfortunately, this seems unlikely. The major stumbling block to the use of HLA typing is that around 20% of the general population carry the exact same HLA subtype, and yet experience none of the symptoms associated with narcolepsy. Furthermore, there are patients with narcolepsy who do not carry the HLA-DQB1*0602 gene.

- *Hypocretin levels:* If the use of HLA subtypes is problematic, could narcolepsy be diagnosed by measuring hypocretin levels in CSF? Researchers at the Stamford University School of Medicine have found that hypocretin levels in CSF are a strong indicator of narcolepsy. Over 90% of narcoleptics with symptoms of cataplexy showed undetectably low levels of hypocretin in their CSF compared to normal controls. So, testing for hypocretin levels certainly offers more promise than HLA typing. There is, however, much more we need to understand about the role of hypocretin before this could be used as a convincing diagnostic test. For instance, we have no clear picture regarding the hypocretin levels of those patients who do not experience cataplexy. Also, as the research conducted using narcoleptic dogs suggested, in some cases, patients' problems may be due to the malfunctioning of hypocretin receptors, rather than the lack of hypocretin itself. If this were the case, normal levels of hypocretin would be detected in the CSF, despite the individual having narcolepsy.

Improving treatment

Narcolepsy is a lifelong condition, which, as yet, has no cure. Currently, the recommended treatment includes a combination of:

- *Medication:* the drugs used are either antidepressants or stimulants such as modafinil or Ritalin. All these drugs act on a group of neurotransmitters called monoamines (these include dopamine, serotonin and noradrenaline) rather than on the hypocretin system. So, while they address the symptoms, they do not address the root cause of the disorder
- *Counselling* to help cope with the emotional consequences of having the disorder
- *Behavioural changes* to help the patient manage the condition.

Refining drug treatments

Now that we know that low levels of hypocretin are central in many cases of narcolepsy, scientists are working on developing treatments to supplement hypocretin levels and reduce the symptoms. Correcting hypocretin levels is not, however, straightforward. Drugs that can be given by mouth or injection to correct levels are unstable and are usually broken down before reaching the brain. One possible way to overcome this would be to use high dosages, but this carries greater risks of major side effects and would need to be tested on genetically modified animals to ensure safety. Perhaps a better option would be to create an artificial drug that can penetrate the brain and 'replace' the missing hypocretin, but this will take some considerable time to develop.

Cell transplantation

Although our understanding of the hypocretin deficiency in narcolepsy may help to develop more effective treatments, it is unlikely that this knowledge will enable the process to be reversed, as it seems that the cells that secrete hypocretin are actually destroyed by the immune system. If this proves to be the case, a cure for narcolepsy would need to involve the transplantation of new hypocretin-producing cells into the appropriate area of the hypothalamus. Currently, the techniques for transplanting cells into the brain are being explored in other clinical conditions, for example in Parkinson's disease, but it is likely to be many years before cell transplantation becomes a treatment option for narcolepsy.

Psychology as science → **The use of animals in research**

Much of the research that has looked at the causes of narcolepsy has been conducted using animal populations. While this type of research provides useful insights into possible causes and directions for future research using humans, the findings cannot easily be extrapolated and generalized to humans:

- although there are some basic similarities, the anatomy and physiology of animals and humans are different, particularly in relation to brain function. Extrapolation must only be done with caution
- there are significant differences in the sleep patterns of humans and animals
- humans have far greater cognitive abilities than animals, which allows them to think about experiences and explain experiences in ways that animals simply cannot. These cognitive abilities may mediate and moderate the patterns of sleep. For example, if an experience is seen as worrying, the worry itself may affect the duration and quality of sleep.

There are also important ethical issues involved when using animals in research studies, and the breeding of genetically modified animals is a highly emotive topic, which requires a careful cost–benefit analysis before it can be justified.

👁 Sleepwalking

Sleepwalking (SW), or **somnambulism** as it is technically known, is a sleep disorder belonging to the parasomnia group. According to the National Sleep Foundation (www.sleepfoundation.org), SW is experienced by between 1 and 15% of the general population. It is most commonly found among children, with estimates suggesting that around 30% of 5- to 12-year-olds experience occasional SW episodes, while 1–5% sleepwalk on a regular basis. Although SW normally disappears by adolescence, around 3% of adults suffer from the disorder. Adult sufferers experience more frequent SW episodes than children, and adult episodes are often related to times of stress. SW in old age is rare and is usually associated with other age-related disorders.

There is a sense of mystery associated with SW that has led to its frequent appearance in art and literature. In Shakespeare's *Macbeth*, for instance, Lady Macbeth sleepwalks because of overwhelming guilt and insanity. Bellini wrote an opera called *La Somnambula* ('The Sleep-walker') and SW even featured in the Harry Potter film *Harry Potter and the Prisoner of Azkaban* when Harry used SW as an excuse to explain why he was out of bed after hours.

Behaviour during sleepwalking episodes

It is unusual for SW episodes to occur more than once a night, and when they do, it is generally during the first third of the night (between 11pm and 1am) in the deeper phases of NREM sleep. During an episode, the sleepwalker arises from bed and performs activities that are usually performed during the day. These may be as simple as sitting up or walking around, but are sometimes quite complex, such as eating, bathing, dressing, texting, emailing, walking the dog, dancing or cooking a meal. SW episodes almost always involve actions that are very familiar, and typically last anything from a few seconds to as long as 30 minutes. Sometimes SW is accompanied by sleep-talking, in which the sleep-walker produces meaningless streams of words. Although the sleep-walker's eyes are open during the episode, they are not conscious, and when woken, either in the morning or during an episode – which is not dangerous as once thought, although it may leave the sleeper feeling a little disorientated – they have no memory of the events that took place during the episode.

Consequences of sleepwalking

The consequences of SW are not generally dangerous, particularly when SW occurs in a familiar environment, and sleepwalkers are generally able to negotiate their way successfully around objects and open and shut doors. When, however, they are in an unfamiliar setting, there may be some degree of danger as sleepwalkers do not respond to their immediate environment and accidents can easily happen. In extreme cases, in which the sufferer experiences one or more episodes a night, SW may have a severe effect on the individual's life, particularly in terms of their relationship with other family members.

Causes of sleepwalking

Psychodynamic explanation

Early explanations, driven by the Freudian perspective, suggested that SW was the result of a dreamer acting out a dream. For example, the Society for Science and the Public (1954), concluded that SW was the result of:

> repression of hostile feelings against the father caused the patients to react by acting out in a dream world with sleepwalking, the distorted fantasies they had about all authoritarian figures, such as fathers, officers and stern superiors.

An alternative psychodynamic explanation was proposed, based on the observation that the behaviour of sleepwalkers looks as if it has real purpose. This suggested that SW represented a desire to sleep where the person slept as a child.

As always with psychodynamic explanations of behaviour, these hypotheses are not easily tested in any objective way. Biological evidence, however, challenges the view that SW is the acting out of dreams and desires. SW occurs during NREM (stages 3 and 4) phases of sleep and not during REM sleep. Dreams are predominantly associated with REM sleep (Chapter 3) and it is physically impossible for sleepers to move around during REM sleep as the muscles of the body are paralysed. Dreams cannot be acted out during SW.

Biological explanations

Various biological explanations have been put forward to explain SW behaviour.

Incomplete arousal

EEG recordings of brain activity during SW, collected in sleep laboratories, show a mix of slow delta waves, characteristic of NREM, mixed with beta waves, which are found in waking states. This suggests that there may be a problem with the systems that control brain arousal, with the sleepwalker being partially, but not completely, aroused.

Delayed brain development

The observation that children generally grow out of SW has led to the suggestion that the neural circuits responsible for controlling the sleep–waking cycle may be underdeveloped in those who sleepwalk (Oliviero, 2008). However, although delayed neural development may explain some aspects of the disorder, it cannot explain why, for instance, adults are more likely to sleepwalk when stressed.

Functional problems in the raphe nuclei

Evidence has also been found suggesting that SW may be caused by a failure of the serotonin system in the raphe nuclei, an area of the brain that is central to the control of the sleep–waking cycle (Hafeez and Kalinowski, 2007). In particular, the raphe nuclei seem to be involved in the regulation of NREM (see Chapter 3).

Genes

There are a number of lines of evidence that suggest that genes may play an important role in SW. Family studies show that SW behaviour tends to run in families, and the likelihood of SW increases to 45% if one parent is affected and 60% if both parents are affected (Lavie et al., 2002).

A study aimed at uncovering the specific genetic involvement in SW (Lecendreux et al., 2003) examined the set of genes known as HLA, discussed above in relation to narcolepsy. These genes provide the information needed to allow the body to create immune cells, and have been linked to a number of other sleep disorders including narcolepsy. Sixty sleepwalkers and 60 matched controls were examined, and it was found that the sleepwalkers were 3.5 times more likely to have a subtype of the gene HLA-DQB1 than controls. This figure was even higher when there was a history of SW in the family.

To uncover the degree to which genes contribute to SW, a large-scale questionnaire study, involving 11,220 pairs of twins, was conducted in Finland. The study found a concordance rate of 0.55 in monozygotic twins and 0.35 among dizygotic twins. The researchers concluded that the tendency to SW is more than 50% genetically based (Hublin et al., 1997). Large-scale studies such as this are extremely valuable. It is only by using such a large sample of the target population that we can sort out the extent to which behaviour has a genetic basis and the extent to which behaviour can be attributed to environmental or psychological causes.

Diathesis-stress model

SW, in common with other sleep conditions, is a complex disorder, influenced by both genes and environment. There is clear evidence for a significant genetic involvement, yet it seems that genes can only account for about 50% of the incidence of SW. It may be that genes predispose a person to SW but there has to be a precipitating factor. This has yet to be conclusively identified. It may be any one of a number of factors that have been shown to increase NREM sleep stages, such as sleep deprivation, excessive tiredness, high bodily temperature, stress, psychiatric conditions, or drug or alcohol use.

Is sleepwalking behaviour under an individual's control?

In Chapter 1 we discussed some issues in relation to consciousness and awareness. There is a clear distinction between primary consciousness or basic awareness, and higher order consciousness or self-awareness. In waking life, we show this higher order consciousness, but in states such as dreams, we are demonstrating only basic awareness without self-awareness. Can we locate SW within concepts of consciousness?

This is not straightforward. There appears to be only a simple reactivity to the environment as the movements seem automatic rather than carefully planned. This is not the basic awareness or primary consciousness that we might see in animals, but an even more basic level of consciousness, with certainly no self-awareness. Sleepwalking occurs in the deeper stages of NREM sleep, stages usually associated with deep sleep and complete loss of conscious awareness. So we can conclude that in genuine SW, only a rudimentary consciousness is present, with certainly no self-awareness.

There is much discussion and excitement in the media about crimes that occur when people appear to be SW. This is an area of interest particularly for the legal profession, as a person cannot be held responsible for their actions if they are not conscious of them. The severity of punishment is also based on the level of responsibility. Examples of SW cases include Steven Steinberg who, in 1981, was accused of killing his wife in the middle of the night; Scott Falater who, in 1997, stabbed his wife 44 times; Brain Thomas, who killed his wife while dreaming she was an intruder; and Kenneth Parks, who drove to his mother-in-law's house, some 14 miles away, and stabbed her, while claiming to be still asleep. If these were genuine cases of SW, the defendants would not have been conscious and self-aware of their actions, and so not responsible for them. Unfortunately, SW is easy to fake, so the only time the 'sleep-walking' defence might be accepted is when there is a clearly documented medical history of a SW disorder.

Defences in these types of case may also suggest that the crimes are the result of the individual acting out a dream, but because SW normally occurs during NREM phases of sleep, it would not be possible for these crimes to be explained in this way. As pointed out above, dreams mostly occur in REM sleep when body muscles are paralysed and SW would be impossible. There is, however, a particular and rare form of SW in which patients do seem to act out their dreams. This disorder, known as REM sleep behavioural disorder (RSBD), tends to occur in later life (age 50+) and affects more men than women.

Causes of REM sleep behavioural disorder

There has been relatively little research into REM sleep behavioural disorder (RSBD), but two possible explanations have been put forward:

1 *Genes:* RSBD appears to have a strong genetic component, with 85% of male sufferers having been found to have a HLA–DQwl genetic marker (Schenck and Mahowald, 1996).
2 *Damage to the magnocellular nucleus,* which allows movement during REM sleep: Normally during REM sleep the body is paralysed, specifically to prevent people acting out their dreams and harming themselves or others. The mechanism that controls this is associated with the neurotransmitter acetylcholine and involves a region of the brain called the magnocellular nucleus. This normally sends signals to the spinal cord that prevent motor pathways being activated and so results in paralysis. It has been suggested that, in RSBD, damage to the magnocellular nucleus may cause this blocking action to fail, so allowing the sleeper to move around during REM sleep and physically act out their dreams (Culebras and Moore, 1989).

So are people with RSBD responsible for their actions? Dreams are a state in which the dreamer behaves in complex ways, reacting to the world around, that is, showing primary consciousness. However, there is no self-awareness; with rare exceptions (see Chapter 5) we are not aware we are dreaming while we are dreaming. If the actions carried out in RSBD are effectively dreams, then we cannot assume that the person has self-awareness. The science would suggest that they are not responsible for their actions. Of course, in a legal setting, this defence would only be viable if there was an established clinical history of RSBD.

Summary

- Sleep disorders are divided into dyssomnias, where problems with the amount or timing of sleep lead to daytime sleepiness, and parasomnias, where problems associated with sleep do not lead to daytime sleepiness. Insomnia and narcolepsy are dyssomnias, while sleepwalking and REM sleep behavioural disorder are parasomnias.
- Insomnia can be divided into primary and secondary insomnia. In primary insomnia, there is no identifiable medical or psychological condition that might lead to the symptoms. Secondary insomnia can be linked to such identifiable conditions.
- Primary insomnia has been associated with high levels of anxiety and arousal, poor sleep habits, abnormalities of sleep control systems, and there is some evidence for a genetic involvement.
- Secondary insomnia can be caused by a range of medical, neurological and psychological conditions. It is also associated with stimulants such as caffeine and tobacco, and other sleep disorders such as apnoea and sleepwalking.
- Other factors that predispose to insomnia include genetic factors, personality, age and gender.
- Individuals have particular chronotypes. At the extremes, morning types (larks) are more alert in the early morning, while evening types (owls) are more alert in the evening. Chronotype is determined by the characteristics of the internal body clocks controlling the circadian sleep–waking cycle.
- Precipitating factors for insomnia include environmental stressors, life events, diet, drugs and alcohol. Perpetuating factors include sleeping pills, alcohol and nicotine.

- Hypersomnia is a rare dyssomnia characterized by excessive daytime sleepiness. It may be related to genetic abnormalities of the sleep–waking system. It can also be secondary to brain damage, infections, medical conditions such as depression or encephalitis, or various medications.
- Narcolepsy is a dramatic disorder whose symptoms include excessive daytime sleepiness, cataplexy, hallucinations and sleep paralysis. It appears to be a REM sleep-related disorder, as sufferers move directly into REM at the start of sleep rather than having a phase of light NREM beforehand.
- There is strong evidence for genetic factors in narcolepsy, probably involving control of the brain neurotransmitter hypocretin. There is no fully effective treatment for narcolepsy, although stimulant drugs can help.
- Sleepwalking occurs in the deep stages of NREM sleep, and is most common in young children. EEG recording suggests that sleepwalkers show a mixed deep sleep/arousal pattern of brain activity. This may indicate incomplete control of sleep mechanisms that may be inherited, as there is clear evidence that sleepwalking runs in families.
- REM sleep behavioural disorder (RSBD) is a rare condition affecting older people. They seem to be acting out dreams, and it may reflect a breakdown in the normal brain systems paralysing the body musculature during REM sleep.

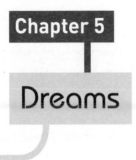

Chapter 5

Dreams

◉ Introduction

> We are such stuff as dreams are made on, rounded with a little
> sleep! (Shakespeare, *The Tempest*, Act 4, scene 1)

The phenomenon of dreams has fascinated people since the earliest
times, with frequent references from the earliest recorded writings. For
instance, in the Bible, Joseph's ability to interpret the dreams of the
pharaoh leads ultimately to the liberation of the people of Israel. Dreams
are clearly a special state of awareness. Although we cannot recall all our
dreams in the morning, we know that, in the dreams we do remember, we
are 'conscious', responding to people and situations in much the same
way we do when awake. This means that dreams represent at least
primary consciousness, the basic awareness and reactivity that we see in
animals (this was discussed in Chapter 1). However, in the dream we are
not aware that we are dreaming, that is, we do not have 'self-awareness',
the higher order consciousness that characterizes our waking behaviour.

Dreams are undoubtedly a fascinating phenomenon, but they have
proved remarkably difficult to study from a scientific perspective. There
is one simple reason for this; dreams are part of our individual, subjective experience. No one else has access to the content of our dreams, and
they only know we have had them because we tell them. The methods of
science rely on objective measurement or assessment, and have few techniques for dealing with subjective experience.

Another problem with research into dreams is that the earliest systematic theories were based in the psychodynamic approach of psychologists
such as Freud and Jung, as discussed in Chapter 1 in relation to consciousness. For most of the twentieth century, psychodynamic psychology and

scientific experimental psychology were mutually incompatible. Freud, for example, was seen as non-scientific, in that his ideas were not easily testable using scientific techniques.

However, given that dreams are part of our subjective experience, it may be that they cannot be studied using scientific techniques. In which case, it would be sensible to use any methods available, even if those include the non-scientific techniques of Freud and other psychodynamic theorists.

In this chapter, we will cover:
- The nature of dreams
- Psychological theories of dreaming
- Neurobiological theories of dreaming
- Lucid dreaming

It is important to remember that dreams have other characteristics than simply their content. In Chapter 3, we reviewed the pioneering discoveries on sleep characteristics of Aserinsky and Kleitman in the 1950s. Their discovery of the different phases of sleep, REM and NREM, was followed up by Dement, who demonstrated conclusively that REM sleep was associated with dreaming; participants woken up during REM sleep reported dreaming 80% of the time, whereas those woken during NREM sleep reported dreaming only 10–15% of the time. In addition, while REM dreams usually had a narrative or storyline with vivid imagery, NREM dreams tended to be less coherent and less vivid. The association between REM sleep and dreaming seemed so strong that REM sleep is still sometimes referred to as 'dreaming sleep'.

Although the association is not perfect, as dreaming also occurs in NREM sleep, it does suggest strongly that there is a special relationship between REM sleep and dreaming. As we shall see later, some theories of dreaming, referred to as **neurobiological theories**, try to explain both the neurophysiological characteristics of REM sleep and the imagery of dreams. However, you should not think that REM sleep and dreaming are the same thing; REM sleep is a physiological state, it is defined by a particular pattern of EEG arousal, activation of specific parts of the brain, eye movements and loss of muscle tone. All these characteristics can be measured objectively. Dreams are very different; they are subjective and cannot be measured objectively. So be careful that you do not fall into the trap of seeing the two terms, REM sleep and dreams, as referring to the same thing. They are not interchangeable or **isomorphic**. In simple terms, isomorphic means that talking about REM sleep would be the same as talking about dreams. It would also mean that dreams occurred whenever we entered REM sleep, and only when we were in REM sleep. As we have seen, this is not the case.

The nature of dreams

Dement's original observations on the nature of dreams have largely stood the test of time. They occur predominantly in REM sleep and occur in real time; that is, the experience of time in the dream is the same as it would be in the real world. Dreams often have a narrative structure, even if the story they tell has bizarre elements. They can be highly emotional or, as with nightmares, unpleasant and anxiety provoking. It is also a feature of dreams that they often contain aspects of the previous day's events, or references to current concerns and worries.

Because the content of dreams can be identified and usually related to the person's life experiences, there have always been enthusiastic attempts to give them meaning. In the biblical reference earlier, Joseph interpreted the pharaoh's dreams in terms of the coming seven plagues of Egypt. Nowadays, any bookshop will have several books helping you to interpret your own dreams. Of course, they are all likely to give different meanings to the same dream content, and it can be difficult to see anything systematic in the analysis of dream symbolism. One non-controversial approach is to provide a general categorization of dreams, such as the one produced by Hunt in 1989. He classified dreams into several categories on the basis of their content:

- Personal dreams – with content of direct personal relevance
- Medical dreams – with content related to health
- Spiritual dreams
- Prophetic dreams – with content that can be interpreted as predicting future events
- Nightmares
- Lucid dreams – the unusual experience of actually being conscious and self-aware during a dream.

This type of classification emphasizes that although all our dreams are unique, there are consistencies in content. However, even though we can classify dreams into general categories, we still need to explain the precise meaning of the unique dreams that people have.

👁 Psychological theories of dreaming

The first category of dream theories we shall look at is the purely psychological approach, best exemplified by the influential work of Sigmund Freud.

Freud's theory of dreaming

> The interpretation of dreams is the royal road to a knowledge of the unconscious activities of the mind. (Freud, [1900]1955)

For Freud, a dream represented the expression of desires that have been repressed into the unconscious mind. These desires, often sexual or aggressive, would be too disturbing for the dreamer if they were aware of them. Even in the dream, these urges have to be disguised, that is, the function of the dream is to allow some expression of these repressed urges, but in a form that does not disturb the dreamer. For the Freudian therapist, the dream therefore has a **manifest content**, which is the dream imagery as reported by the dreamer. For the analyst, though, this manifest content is only the surface, and needs to be interpreted by the analyst in order to reveal the deeper or **latent content**. This latent content is, then, a direct reflection of the repressed urges. The therapist can use the latent content, once revealed, to help the client come to terms with their repressed drives.

The dream work

The conversion of the underlying and threatening impulses and desires into the manifest content of the dream involves the **dream work**. This is controlled by the ego, and involves various processes, including displacement, condensation and representability:

- *Displacement* occurs when the true object of the impulses or desires is converted into another person or object in the manifest content. An example given by Freud concerned a client who reported that in her dream she strangled a little white dog, Freud concluded, after analysis, that the dog represented the client's sister-in-law. The sister-in-law happened to have very pale skin and Freud's client had a difficult relationship with her. Actually dreaming of strangling her sister-in-law would have been too traumatic for the client, so the dream work displaced the feelings onto a dream symbol that was more acceptable to the dreamer.

- *Condensation* describes the way a particular symbol in the manifest content of the dream can represent several different latent impulses or anxieties. For instance, dreaming of one powerful figure may represent the dreamer's father as well as other powerful people in the dreamer's life. These various figures are condensed into the single symbol reported by the dreamer.
- *Representability* refers to the way abstract ideas might come to be represented by real and concrete objects and symbols in a dream. For example, anxieties about power or authority in general may be represented in the dream by a single person such as a father or similar authority figure.

These processes allow threatening impulses – the latent content – to be expressed in the manifest content of the dream. If accurately expressed in the dream, these thoughts and impulses would be too threatening for the dreamer. According to Freud, the role of the analyst, using their knowledge of the dream world, is to interpret the manifest content of the dream and reveal the underlying latent content. This would allow them to help the client come to terms with these underlying anxieties.

During his work, Freud developed a dictionary of dream symbols. Using the many hundreds of dreams reported by his clients, and also his knowledge of the cultural symbols found in fairy stories, mythology, jokes and so on, he gradually developed his dream vocabulary. The best-known example would be his proposal that dreaming of flying represented sexual intercourse, while rockets and boats represented the penis.

However, Freud was also very down to earth and was happy to acknowledge that sometimes the manifest content had no latent meaning. As he put it, 'sometimes a cigar is just a cigar'. It is important to note that Freud also accepted that dream imagery was often dominated by the previous day's events, and we should note that this observation is now a critical part of many modern psychological and neurobiological models of dreaming.

Evaluation

We have already mentioned that the key problem in all models of dreaming is the subjective nature of dream imagery. There is no scientific way of checking whether people's reports of their dreams are accurate. This is a particular problem with theories that focus on the actual dream imagery itself, such as Freud's. Freud also depends absolutely on his interpretation of the dream imagery and this also cannot be validated scientifically. An example of this is the split with Carl Jung. Freud and Jung were colleagues in the early years of the psychoanalytic movement, but Jung eventually disagreed with key aspects of Freud's psychodynamic theory and developed his own school of psychoanalysis. One area where he developed very different ideas to Freud was in the meaning and interpretation of dreams, and there is no easy way to decide which of them is correct.

One way to assess the validity of Freud's theory of dreaming would be to see how successful dream analysis has been in helping clients undergoing psychoanalytic therapy. Unfortunately, systematic and controlled studies of the effectiveness of dream analysis are rare, and what we have in the main are the personal accounts of case studies.

As with many of Freud's ideas, his model of the functions of dreams is easy to dismiss as non-scientific and non-testable, but it has had a tremendous influence on cultural and social attitudes to dreams and dream imagery. Even the fiercest critic of Freud would have to admit that, when thinking about dreams, it is hard to ignore Freud's interpretation of their symbolism, even if deep down we don't believe in the underlying model.

Problem-solving theories

It is a common observation that dream imagery reflects current events in the person's life, and as we shall see later, some neurobiological theories emphasize that the brain is integrating the day's events with previous stored memories. Another approach to this aspect of dream imagery is to see the dream as a time when the brain is actively trying to solve problems in the person's life, and to come up with solutions. This is linked to the popular idea that dreams can be creative, although evidence for this is largely anecdotal. For instance, the chemist Kekule is said to have discovered the chemical nature of the benzene ring when stimulated by a dream of a snake biting its own tail. One of Coleridge's most famous poems, the *Rubaiyat of Omar Khayyam*, was said to have come to him in a dream.

A more systematic approach was taken by Cartwright (1984). She proposed that dreams are important in helping us to cope emotionally with major life stresses. For instance, she compared the dream imagery of divorced women, one group of whom were very depressed after the divorce, while the other group were better adjusted. Cartwright found that the dreams of the depressed group were shorter and made little or no reference to the divorce or to marriage. The dreams of the non-depressed group were longer and contained imagery reflecting the negative emotions produced by the divorce. Cartwright concluded that dreams could be an adaptive response to stressful situations, and dealing with the situations in the dream allowed for a better emotional adjustment to life in general. She noted that as the mood of the depressed group of divorced women improved, their dreams too began to reflect the feelings aroused by the divorce. Cartwright would argue that this processing of negative emotions in the dream was actually helping to improve their waking mood state.

Neurobiological theories of dreaming

Psychological theories of dreams pay great attention to the actual dream imagery and the meanings it may have. This approach reaches its climax in the work of Freud. In contrast, the neurobiological approach, while acknowledging that the key characteristic of dreams is dream imagery, pays less attention, if any, to any meaning the imagery may have. These approaches focus on the brain activity that we know occurs during dreaming. In Chapter 3, we briefly discussed the relationship between REM sleep and dreaming, and neurobiological theories focus on the particular pattern of brain activity associated with REM sleep, and from this try to explain the occurrence of dreams.

We have already seen that the brain is highly active during REM sleep, with energy consumption not far short of waking levels. It is therefore no surprise that during REM sleep, high levels of neural activity can be recorded in the cortex (the higher levels of brain function) and in the subcortical and brainstem regions. Neurobiological theories propose that these patterns of neural activity reflect information processing during REM sleep, with dream imagery as a byproduct of this activity. However, as with Freud and other psychodynamic approaches, there is no generally agreed view on exactly what this information processing might represent.

Crick and Mitchison's reverse learning theory

Crick and Mitchison's (1983) **reverse learning theory of dreaming** (incidentally, Francis Crick, together with James Watson, won the

Nobel prize for describing the role of DNA in genetics) sees REM sleep as the time when the brain is sorting through the information received during the day and eliminating what are called 'parasitic' thoughts. The cortex receives a huge amount of information during our waking activities, and for efficient functioning, it needs to dispose of information it doesn't need. These unwanted thoughts or memories are represented as neural connections in the cortex. During REM sleep, we know that the connections between the cortex and subcortical structures are highly active, with the cortex 'bombarded' by signals from subcortical structures. The reverse learning model proposes that this activity represents the elimination of the parasitic cortical connections and the unwanted memories they represent. Dream imagery is made up of these parasitic memories as they are being eliminated. The term 'reverse learning' refers to the fact that material acquired, or learned, during the day is now being erased.

This theory is based on the patterns of brain activity during REM sleep and on a number of computer simulations of how memory is organized in the brain. Apart from this, there is very little direct evidence for or against the proposal. Crick and Mitchison (1983) do use two examples from the animal kingdom to support their model. The primitive mammal echidna (the spiny anteater) and the dolphin appear to have little or no REM sleep. According to the Crick and Mitchison model, they are therefore missing out on the opportunity to filter out unwanted or parasitic memories. However, they do have relatively enlarged cortical areas, and Crick and Mitchison suggest that this is because they need to store the unwanted memories that in other species are disposed of during REM sleep. This is very indirect evidence and it can also be pointed out that humans have an enlarged cortex, but we also have REM sleep, so we cannot argue that if you have one, you don't need the other.

Finally, and to emphasize that even the most neurobiological theory cannot ignore dream imagery, it is a problem for the reverse learning approach that many dreams are organized and coherent. If dreams were simply a byproduct of the random elimination of parasitic memories, then we would expect them to be fragmented and bizarre. Later on, Crick and Mitchison did, in fact, restrict their ideas to dreams that were fragmented and incoherent.

Hobson and McCarley's activation-synthesis theory

Hobson and McCarley (1977) based their ideas about dreaming on many experimental studies on the nature of REM sleep in humans and animals. In REM sleep, brainstem areas are highly active, and the pathways from the reticular formation to the cortex are very active. Consequently, widespread regions of the cortex are aroused, including areas specialized for the processing of visual and auditory input and also areas involved in the control of movement. The activation of sensory and motor areas during REM sleep accounts for dream imagery. If visual and auditory areas are activated during REM sleep, we will see things and hear things. If movement areas are activated, we will experience the sensation of movement, for example walking or running. If the area involved in the control of balance is activated, the dream may include the sensation of falling.

One key issue, of course, is why don't we act out these actions? During REM sleep, in fact, a 'gate' at the top of the spinal cord closes so that we are effectively paralysed. Impulses from the movement control centres in the cortex cannot pass down the spinal cord and out to the muscles of the body. Some rare studies have manipulated this gate in cats, and they have demonstrated that if the gate is open during REM sleep, cats will act out complicated sequences of movements, such as hunting or playing, even though they are in REM sleep.

The **activation-synthesis theory of dreams** explains dream imagery through the brain activation during REM sleep. The synthesis part accounts for the structure of dreams. Hobson and McCarley (1977) propose that the brain has an innate tendency to organize material, and will automatically try to impose a structure on the sights, sounds and movements activated during REM sleep. As recent events during waking would have only recently been stored, they would be very accessible. They are therefore likely to form part of the images activated during REM sleep, and will therefore feature prominently in the dreams that we experience.

The activation-synthesis model relies heavily on the brain's natural tendency to impose structure on the memories, sensations and movements aroused during REM sleep. However, it also argues that this may not happen. In this way, the model can account for both coherent dreams with a clear narrative structure, and also for bizarre and fragmented dreams. Although this can look like a strength, it is also a weakness, as it means we cannot use the characteristics of the dream as a way of testing the model. This is not to say the model is therefore wrong, simply that it is hard to test in a controlled scientific way. The main strength of the model is that it is based on a comprehensive knowledge of the patterns of brain electrical activity during REM sleep , and uses these to account for dream imagery in a way that seems intuitively plausible. It is broader in scope than the reverse learning theory of dreams and is very much embedded in the neurophysiology of REM sleep. In similar fashion to the reverse learning theory, though, it sees dreams as essentially byproducts of brain activity, and therefore essentially meaningless.

More recently, Hobson (2002) has developed the activation-synthesis model into a general theory of REM sleep, NREM sleep, dreaming and consciousness. Although the details are beyond the scope of this book, in brief, Hobson's AIM model tries to locate states of awareness along three dimensions:

- A – *Activation:* the level of brain arousal
- I – *Input:* whether information is entering the brain from external sources, that is, the environment, or is internal – generated by brain systems themselves
- M – *Modulation:* whether the most active pathways in the brain are monoaminergic, for example using the neurotransmitter noradrenaline, or cholinergic – using the neurotransmitter acetylcholine. Different pathways are involved in different aspects of information processing in the brain.

In Hobson's view, REM (dreaming) sleep, for example, represents a high level of brain activation, an internal source of input, and brain modulation is via cholinergic pathways. The waking alert state is associated with high levels of brain arousal, an external source of information input, and monoaminergic modulation. Deep NREM sleep is then characterized by low levels of brain activation, low levels of internal inputs, and cholinergic modulation. Then, as we move from REM to NREM sleep and finally to waking, so the brain shifts along the three dimensions.

Hobson's AIM model is a useful way of conceptualizing the key characteristics of REM and NREM sleep. He also tries to account for other altered states of awareness such as hallucinations, but whether the model remains simply another way of describing states or whether it can actually help to understand and explain them remains to be seen.

A synthesis: Revonsuo's threat simulation theory

Theories of dreaming derived from the neurobiological approach see dreams as essentially a byproduct (or epiphenomenon) of brain activity during REM sleep. They do not believe that dreams have any function in their own right. Psychological approaches, such as those emphasizing problem solving, do give dreams an important function, but evidence is inconclusive as to whether they genuinely help us to cope with life's problems. However, there is no doubt that our dream imagery often incorporates elements from our current concerns and anxieties.

Revonsuo (2000) proposes a biological approach to dreaming, in that it emphasizes the evolutionary function of dreaming. But it differs from the neurobiological models outlined above, in that it has a central role for dream imagery. The **threat simulation theory of dreams**, or 'evolutionary hypothesis' as Revonsuo also calls it, is made up of six propositions (Revonsuo, 2000):

1 Dream content is not random or disorganized; rather it is an organized simulation of the actual perceptual world.
2 Dream consciousness is specialized for the simulation of threatening events. From this proposition, Revonsuo made three predictions:
   - Threats will be overrepresented in dreams
   - Severe or life-threatening events will be included in dreams more frequently than in waking life
   - If triggered by real-life events, the threat simulation mechanism should generate rehearsals of ancient threats, for example animal attacks, physical aggression, more easily than modern threats, for example traffic accidents, explosions.
3 Exposure to threatening events in real life activates the threat simulation mechanism.
4 The threat simulations produced by the fully activated system in dreams are perceptually and behaviourally realistic rehearsals of threat perception and avoidance. From this, Revonsuo predicted that, when in mortal danger, the dreamer is likely to display reasonable and realistic defensive action in the dream.
5 The perceptual and motor simulations provided by dreams lead to improved performance in real-life threat situations, even when the dream rehearsal is not explicitly remembered.

6 It is reasonable to assume that our ancestors in the environment of evolutionary adaptation over 2 million years ago spent much of their lives exposed to real threats and dangers. The human dream system developed as a means of simulating these threats during sleep and practising ways of dealing with them. If this leads to a better chance of survival in the real world, then such dream mechanisms would provide a 'selective advantage' in Darwinian evolutionary terms and would therefore persist through human evolution. So, although dreams are part of our subjective experience, the brain mechanisms underlying them have provided an evolutionary advantage as dreams improve our chances of surviving in the real world.

This is a fascinating hypothesis, but like all dream models, it is hard to test. Much of the evidence has to come from studies on the content of dreams. Revonsuo reviews this work and claims that most emotions in dreams are negative, that dreams often focus on the misfortunes of life, and that aggression is the most common form of social interaction. Dreams of being chased are also very frequent. He claims that this shows that dreams are biased towards threatening content, which is consistent with our early evolutionary history.

The idea that our threat simulation system is activated by real-world events is supported by studies of post-traumatic stress disorder (PTSD). After experiences such as war, rape and violent attack, the sufferer's dreams often replay the event. However, there is little evidence that these dreams associated with PTSD help the person to cope with the experience, and Neilsen and Germaine (2000) claim that dreams and nightmares associated with PTSD are, in fact, dysfunctional and delay recovery.

Thinking scientifically → Testing theories of dream function

Much of Revonsuo's evidence comes from a number of studies of dream content that have used a coding technique developed by Hall and Van de Castle (1966). However, a number of other similar studies, using the Hall and Van de Castle system as well as others developed subsequently, come to very different conclusions.

Ardito (2000) for instance, points out that while negative emotions may be common in dreams, they vary from the threat-type emphasized by Revonsuo to emotions such as sadness and confusion that are not threat related. Strauch and Meier (1996) found in their study that the most common emotion reported in dreams was joy. Even some of the types of aggression coded in the Hall and Van de Castle system could not be considered as threat related in Revonsuo's terms; for instance the death of someone else in the dream or killing insects and other animals.

In direct opposition to Revonsuo, Zadra and Donderi (2000) claim that dreams of being chased are in fact rare, occurring less than 15% of the time, while themes supposedly very relevant to our ancestors, such as snakes, fire and natural disasters, are equally uncommon. Finally, many dreams contain unrealistic elements such as floating and flying, which are accompanied by pleasant feelings.

Of course, Revonsuo can claim that we live in a very different world and that he does not claim that all dreams are part of the threat simulation system. However, he would predict that there should be a relationship between life-threatening events in the real world and dream imagery of coping with the threat, and possibly some link between dream imagery and successful coping with future threats. In a direct test of this hypothesis, Malcolm-Smith and Solms (2004) did a content analysis on 401 dreams from 100 men and 301 women. They found that only 8.48% of dreams contained realistic life-threatening events and in only one-third of these did a successful escape occur, while 44.58% of the sample had experienced actual life-threatening events in real life. Malcolm-Smith and Solms claim that these findings contradict Revonsuo's threat simulation hypothesis; this would predict that threat-related imagery should be common in dream reports and would be associated with coping attempts. In addition, real-life threats should increase the activation of the threat simulation system and lead to more threat-related dreams.

The debate over Revonsuo's model exemplifies some of the frustrations of studying dreams scientifically. Dream imagery may vary with gender, age and culture – the Malcolm-Smith and Solms study, for instance, was carried out in South Africa, a more violent society than the UK. Domhoff (1996) concluded that male dreams contained more aggressive imagery than female dreams, although Malcolm-Smith and Solms found no gender differences in their study. We have already noted that systems for categorizing dream content, such as Hall and Van de Castle's, must be used carefully as people may use terms such as 'aggressive' in different ways. This means that studies of dream content can produce very different results, and theorists may then carefully select the studies they quote in order to support their hypotheses (Malcolm-Smith and Solms, 2004).

👁 Lucid dreaming

There is no doubt that, by any definition, 'dreaming' is an altered state of consciousness or awareness. During the dream, we have primary consciousness, in the sense that we are aware of what is going on, we respond to situations, events and people. It is very different to waking because we are not aware we are dreaming until we wake up, that is, in the dream we do not have self-awareness. Although we sometimes have a confused period just after waking when we may not be sure whether we are still in the dream, two minutes later we know we are awake and that we were dreaming. We can clearly distinguish two states of awareness.

When we are dreaming, we are generally unresponsive to the world outside, although we may incorporate some sounds or stimuli into a dream. This was demonstrated in the original studies of Dement and Kleitman (1957); if they dripped water onto a participant in REM sleep, they often reported dreams involving water when they awoke. By and large, though, dreams seem to be very separate from waking behaviour and awareness.

However, in 1985, Stephen LaBerge reported a study on what he called **lucid dreaming**. In lucid dreams, the dreamer does become aware that they are dreaming during the dream. In addition, they can exercise some control over what happens in the dream, to the extent that they can alter storylines in ways that suit them. Ever since dream research took off in the 1950s, people had reported the phenomenon of lucid dreaming, but sleep researchers were extremely sceptical that such things could happen – if you do not yourself experience lucid dreams, it is a very bizarre phenomenon to imagine. So finally LaBerge, who had been a lucid dreamer since the age of five, worked out a way to demonstrate lucid dreaming scientifically.

He knew that in his lucid dreams he could control movements of his eyes and hands. So, when wired up in a sleep laboratory that recorded his EEG and eye movements, he waited until he entered a phase of lucid dreaming and then deliberately moved his eyes to follow movements of his fingers. In REM sleep, this should be impossible, as the rapid eye movements observed in REM sleep are essentially random. When the researchers checked the eye movement records for LaBerge, they found that controlled eye movements had occurred exactly when they had observed his fingers moving. EEG recordings confirmed that he was in

REM sleep at the time. This was clear evidence that LaBerge had control over his eye and finger movements during REM sleep, and this helped to establish lucid dreaming as a genuine phenomenon.

In fact, there was good evidence earlier that lucid dreaming was a genuine phenomenon. Keith Hearne, a PhD student at Hull University, studied one participant, Alan Worsley, who may have been the first to demonstrate lucid dreaming in the sleep laboratory (Blackmore, 2003). Hearne and Worsley decided that Worsley would move his eyes left to right eight times in succession whenever he entered a phase of lucid dreaming. When he checked the eye movement recordings, Hearne identified these regular movements in the eye movement recordings, and found that they occurred in the middle of phases of REM sleep.

The original findings of LaBerge and Hearne have been replicated many times, and we now have a fairly complete picture of lucid dreaming (Blackmore, 2003):

- Lucid dreams can be variable in length but on average last about two minutes
- They tend to occur in the early morning
- Around 50% of people have experienced at least one lucid dream, while about 20% have at least one every month
- The frequency of lucid dreaming does not correlate with variables such as age, gender or personality characteristics
- People who have lucid dreams tend to report more out-of-body experiences than non-lucid dreamers.

Although we do know a great deal about lucid dreaming, we still do not have an explanation for it or a description of the underlying brain mechanisms. However, it is possible that other observations may shed some light on the mechanisms of lucid dreaming.

It has been observed that some patients with brain damage to the pathways connecting the higher frontal parts of the brain with deeper lying structures of the limbic system report losing the capacity to dream. EEG recording shows that they still have REM sleep (you may remember that key circuits controlling REM and NREM sleep are located in the brainstem, buried deep within the brain and not affected by this brain damage). Supporting evidence comes from historical accounts of patients with schizophrenia. A standard treatment for schizophrenia before the introduction of antipsychotic drugs in the early 1950s was the frontal lobotomy. This operation involved cutting the pathways connecting the frontal lobes with the limbic system, very similar to the brain damage just described. The operation did not target the specific symptoms of schizophrenia but did reduce arousal, producing patients who were much easier to manage. However, the interesting observation from our point of view is that a large majority of these lobotomy patients reported that they no longer had dreams. It seems that disconnecting the frontal areas (frontal cortex) from the rest of the brain can eliminate the experience of dreaming, while leaving REM sleep intact. Note that this supports the idea that REM sleep and dreaming are not the same thing, and that you can manipulate one without affecting the other.

Another tentative conclusion is that for dreaming to occur, an intact frontal cortex has to be connected to the rest of the brain. The frontal cortex has many functions, but its most important role is the control of our planning and decision making; how to achieve goals, how to change plans in the light of different outcomes, all the while supervising and coordinating the activities of a range of other brain structures such as the limbic system. The coherent structure of many dreams may be due to this basic supervisory role that the frontal cortex has, and certainly the ability to become 'aware' that one is dreaming in the middle of a dream is something that we would associate with the frontal lobes. They are likely to play key roles in consciousness and self-awareness, as they are the most recently evolved and highly developed areas of the brain, and we saw in Chapter 1 that 'conscious' information processing seems to involve activity in the prefrontal cortex.

Normally, dream consciousness is very different to waking consciousness as most of us are not lucid dreamers and are only fully self-aware when awake. Dreams do engage frontal areas, but not usually the specific regions that are also involved in consciousness and self-awareness in the waking state. For whatever reason, in lucid dreaming this aspect of frontal cortex function is activated, and awareness in dreams that we are actually dreaming, that is, self-awareness, becomes possible. It is interesting that some people can train themselves to become lucid dreamers (LaBerge, 1985). One method introduced by LaBerge was to wake yourself with an alarm in the early morning, write down any dream that you were having, then, as you go back to sleep, keep imagining that you are back in the same dream. According to LaBerge, practise with this technique will lead to the development of lucid dreaming.

Summary

- Dreams are a special state of awareness, reflecting primary consciousness, but because of their subjective nature, they are difficult to study scientifically.
- Psychological approaches to the functions of dreams emphasize the significance of the symbolic content of dreams.
- Freudian theory sees the manifest content of dreams reflecting a latent content that can be anxiety provoking. Manifest content conceals repressed and threatening material that can be interpreted by the therapist through the 'dream work'.
- Problem-solving models see dreams as a way of coping with waking difficulties. So dream content often reflects waking worries.
- Neurobiological approaches see dreams as byproducts of the brain arousal patterns associated with REM sleep.
- The reverse learning model interprets dreams as unwanted material being erased from memory during REM sleep.
- Activation-synthesis theory sees dreams as the inevitable outcome of brain activation during REM sleep in areas controlling vision, hearing, memory and so on. They are produced by the brain's innate tendency to organize information into coherent narratives.
- Threat simulation theory combines psychological and neurobiological approaches as it takes an evolutionary perspective. Dreams actively help in developing coping skills for daytime threats and dangers, and so REM sleep and dreaming have been subject to the selection pressures of evolution.
- Lucid dreaming is the experience of becoming self-aware while dreaming. It allows the dreamer to control dream content and narrative, and is more common than once thought. We have no convincing explanation for lucid dreaming, either psychological or neurobiological, although the involvement of self-awareness points to specific frontal areas of the brain.

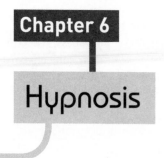

Chapter 6

Hypnosis

👁 Introduction

If someone says the word 'hypnosis', what do you think of? The image that springs to most people's minds, which comes largely from watching films or TV programmes, is of a man swinging a pocket watch to and fro, guiding a participant into a semi-sleep, trance-like state, by softly and slowly saying words such as 'focus on the watch as it gently swings from left to right ... from left to right ... from left to right ... you are now feeling sleepy, very, veeery sleepy'. But can procedures like this really persuade people to carry out the often bizarre commands of the hypnotists we see on the stage or on TV?

Hypnosis has long fascinated both psychologists and the general public because of the dramatic changes in behaviour that it can produce. People who are hypnotized seem to experience the world in a different way. They eat onions and claim they taste of apple, they apparently see things that are not there or fail to see things that are there. They perform behaviours they would not normally be able or willing to do, such as controlling severe pain, showing increased strength, retrieving long-forgotten memories or even running around a stage clucking like a chicken. A key feature is that they do not appear to remember their behaviour when 'awoken' from the hypnotic state. So although they demonstrate primary consciousness in the form of reactive awareness while hypnotized, they do not seem to have self-awareness, in the sense that they are not aware of their hypnotized state during the period they are hypnotized. This is similar to the state of awareness associated with dreams (Chapter 5). So is the hypnotic state a different state of awareness? This is controversial, and there are many other aspects to the study of hypnosis.

In this chapter, we will cover:
- A brief history of hypnosis
- The hypnotic process
- Characteristics of the hypnotic state
- Individual differences in susceptibility to hypnosis
- State theories of hypnosis
- Non-state theories of hypnosis
- State or non-state theories: which view is correct?
- Applications of hypnosis

A brief history of hypnosis

Hypnosis is not a modern phenomenon as it has existed in various forms for centuries. The earliest recorded use of hypnosis was by the cult of Aesculapius, the legendary Greek god of medicine, as long ago as 400 BC. There is also evidence that physicians in ancient Greece and Egypt made use of hypnotic procedures, but it was not until the late eighteenth century that hypnosis attracted serious attention.

Swiss physician Paracelsus (1493–1541) first proposed that diseases could be treated using magnets and the magnetic powers of heavenly bodies. This idea was taken up by the Viennese physician, Franz Anton Mesmer (1734–1815). Mesmer's theory of 'animal magnetism', like Paracelsus's, suggested that illness was caused by an imbalance of magnetic fluids in the body and could be cured by restoring the balance. To treat patients, he would play ethereal music on a glass harmonica, pass his hands across their bodies and wave a magnetic wand over the infected area. During treatment, many patients fell into a hypnotic trance and emerged claiming to feel much better. 'Mesmerism', as it was called, rapidly became popular and was widely used in the treatment of physical and mental disorders. Yet despite the seeming effectiveness of this 'miracle cure', the medical profession remained sceptical. In 1784, the famous American scientist Benjamin Franklin chaired a commission to investigate mesmerism. After considering the evidence, they dismissed the magical element of Mesmer's theory and concluded that there was no scientific basis for Mesmer's animal magnetism.

Although eventually discredited as a healer, Mesmer had clearly demonstrated that the mind could be manipulated by suggestion to produce effects on the body. So powerful were these effects that the practice was resurrected in the nineteenth century and was used to block pain during major surgery (this was before the discovery of the anaesthetic gas ether). It was also during the nineteenth century that Scottish surgeon James Braid changed the name from 'mesmerism' to 'hypnosis', a word derived from the Greek word *hypnos*, meaning 'to sleep'.

Throughout its history, hypnosis has had a difficult relationship with science. There are many who are sceptical of its powers and there is, as yet, no agreement about exactly what it is and how it works, as we will see when we look at the theories of hypnosis later in this chapter.

◉ The hypnotic process

The hypnotic process consists of two phases – an induction phase, which guides the participant into a suggestible frame of mind, followed by a phase in which specific suggestions are made by the hypnotist concerning the way the person should think, feel or behave.

Phase 1: induction

Depending on the participant's personality and the method of induction used, this phase may last anywhere from a few minutes to half an hour. Various induction techniques can be used, all of which share the following common features:

- The goal of focusing attention, filtering out distractions and encouraging the participant to focus on their inner world
- Encouraging participants to be non-analytical in their thinking
- A dependence on the participant wanting to be hypnotized and believing that they can be hypnotized.

The most commonly used hypnotic techniques are:

- *Fixed-gaze induction:* This involves the participant focusing so intently on an object that they tune out all other stimuli. Almost any object can be used – the flame of a candle, a swinging pendulum, or even a single spot on a wall. As the participant focuses, the hypnotist speaks to them in a slow, soft, monotone voice, which lulls the participant into a state of relaxation. This method was widely used in the early days of hypnosis but is not as common today as it does not work as well as some other methods.

- *Progressive relaxation and imagery:* This is the method that is most commonly employed during hypnosis-based therapy. By speaking in a quiet, slow voice, the hypnotist induces a hypnotic trance state. A typical script for inducing hypnosis might be: 'Imagine you are lying on a quiet beach of soft white sand. The sun is shining and you are feeling warm and relaxed and sleepy. You hear the waves gently lapping on the shore and birds calling overhead. You can smell the warm, salt air. Your feel the warmth of the sun on your skin. You are feeling so relaxed. Your eyelids are growing heavy. Very heavy. Your eyes are starting to close.'
- *Rapid induction:* Rapid induction involves overloading the mind with sudden, forceful commands. If the commands are sufficiently forceful and delivered in a sufficiently convincing manner, participants surrender control to the hypnotist. This method is the one most often used by stage hypnotists, as the novelty of standing in front of an audience makes participants feel vulnerable and leaves them more susceptible to the hypnotist's commands.

Although hypnotic induction generally involves some level of relaxation, it is also possible to induce hypnosis during periods of high arousal. For example, in Turkey in the thirteenth century, the Whirling Dervishes, a Sufi branch of Islam, were formed by Jalaleddin Rumi, who used high-energy dancing to produce a trance-like state. Inducing hypnosis during periods of high arousal was also demonstrated in a laboratory by Banyi and Hilgard (1976) who induced a hypnotic, trance-like state while participants cycled on a stationary bicycle.

Phase 2: suggestion

Once a state of hypnotic trance has been induced, the hypnotist begins to verbally communicate suggestions aimed at producing a particular behaviour, thought or feeling. Verbal suggestions are often, but not necessarily, accompanied by appropriate imagery. For example, to reduce the pain of a medical procedure, a hypnotherapist might invoke an image of pain intensity being turned down like the volume on a radio.

Terminating the session

Many people fear that, at the end of a session, they may get 'stuck' in a hypnotized state. However, you can no more get 'stuck' in a hypnotic state than you can get 'stuck' awake or asleep. Hypnosis is a state that naturally gives way to other states of awareness after a while. For practical reasons, most hypnotherapists explicitly end their clients' trances at the end of a session by using direct instructions. If they didn't, the clients would naturally return to full alertness or fall asleep after a short while.

Posthypnotic amnesia

After the session is over, many people appear to suffer from posthypnotic amnesia. This means that they are unable to recall events that have occurred during the session (Bowers and Woody, 1996). These memories have not, however, been permanently erased, they are simply stored in such a way that the conscious mind does not have access to them. If the hypnotist gives a prearranged signal, such as 'When I clap my hand you will remember everything that has taken place', people are usually able to recall what has happened during the session.

Posthypnotic suggestion

It is not only during a session that people act on the directions of the hypnotist. Suggestions can be made during the session that require the participant to act in a certain way when they emerge from their trance. **Posthypnotic suggestion**, as this is known, is often used by stage hypnotists as part of their act, but do posthypnotic suggestions really work? Barnier and McConkey (1998) tested this by giving participants who had been hypnotized 120 prepaid postcards addressed to the researchers. Under hypnosis, the suggestion was made that the participant must post one postcard every day for the next four months. When the researchers counted the cards they had received at the end of the four months, they found that more than half had been sent in accordance with the suggestion. So it seems that posthypnotic suggestion certainly works with some people. We can also see the effectiveness of posthypnotic suggestion in clients who undergo hypnosis in order to change an undesirable behaviour, such as smoking. During hypnosis, the suggestion is made that once they emerge from their trance they should stop smoking, and for many this can be successful.

Self-hypnosis

So far we have only talked about hypnosis induced by a hypnotist. It is, however, perfectly possible for people to self-hypnotize. In fact, some people suggest that all hypnosis is self-hypnosis, since it is not possible to hypnotize someone against their will. Typically, self-hypnosis is induced using progressive relaxation, which involves the use of controlled and regulated breathing, isolation and repetitive chanting.

Characteristics of the hypnotic state

Although the subjective experience of being hypnotized varies to some degree depending on the personality of the volunteer and the method of induction used, there are a number of key characteristics that most people report when undergoing hypnotic procedures.

Focused attention

Although it may look as if hypnosis produces a state that has much in common with sleep, people in a hypnotic trance report that they are actually extremely alert and focused throughout. Their attention narrows and they are easily able to filter out extraneous stimuli. Being fully focused to the exclusion of all else is, of course, not unique to hypnotic trances. There are many everyday states just like this, such as:

- Daydreaming or being lost in thought
- Spending time zoning out in front of the TV
- Being absorbed by an activity, such as listening to music, playing sport or reading
- Driving and not recalling the route taken
- Being absorbed in meditation or relaxation procedures.

In fact, when discussing how they feel, participants often liken the experience to one of daydreaming, or losing oneself in a good book or film.

Extreme suggestibility

Under hypnosis, participants readily obey suggestions and instructions without inhibition or embarrassment, even ones that are bizarre or seemingly impossible. However, a sense of safety and morality remains throughout. Participants report that the feeling they have when obeying commands under hypnosis is very different from the feeling they have when responding to everyday instructions. It seems that rather than feeling in control of the situation and having to make an effort to perform the behaviour, under hypnosis they feel as if they have no control over whether they comply or not. Because of this, the behaviour they produce in response to the command feels effortless.

Relaxation

Typically, people in a hypnotic trance report feeling calm and relaxed. It is probable that under hypnosis their attention is so focused that it filters out everyday worries and doubts.

Suspension of planning

People tend not to plan or initiate activity under hypnosis. Control is given over to the hypnotist.

Performance of atypical behaviour

It is suggested that, under hypnosis, people can perform behaviours they would not usually do in a normal waking state. Although this is true to a limited extent, in every instance so far tested, these are, in fact, behaviours they could actually perform in a normal waking state, although perhaps not as effectively or as easily. Because hypnosis involves attention being highly focused, it is likely that other parts of the mind that are normally used for paying attention can instead be used for paying very close attention to one thing in particular. This can make it look as if people have unusual abilities when under hypnosis.

Thinking scientifically → **Is free will lost under hypnosis?**

People in a hypnotized state report feeling as if they have given up control to the hypnotist. Does this mean that under hypnosis people lose self-awareness and therefore free will? Certainly, stage hypnotists would like us to believe this, but is it actually the case?

One study that set out to test this idea scientifically was carried out by Orne and Evans (1965). They wanted to see whether people could be persuaded into behaving in a morally unacceptable way, that is, would they lose free will and surrender control to the hypnotist. It was suggested to hypnotized participants that they should throw nitric acid, which was in fact only water, into the face of their research assistant – astonishingly, most participants did. This would seem to suggest that participants' behaviour was under the control of the hypnotist.

However, the researchers then tested a second group of participants who were only asked to pretend to be hypnotized – so these participants retained self-awareness and free will. Even more astonishingly, most of these participants also threw the 'acid'. So what was going on? When participants in this and other similar studies were questioned, whether they had been hypnotized or not, all reported that they were completely confident that the hypnotists would not ask them to do anything that would harm either themselves or others. Because of this, they were willing to go along with any suggestion the hypnotist made. So, although it initially looked as if free will had been suspended, these results actually say more about obedience to the authority of the hypnotist than about any loss of free will.

So, it seems that, despite the claims of stage hypnotists, it is neither possible to hypnotize anyone against their will, nor to persuade them into behaving in a way that would go against their moral principles or beliefs. Should a hypnotist make a suggestion to do something that is obviously dangerous or wrong, it is likely that the hypnotized person would either become fully alert or simply ignore the suggestion.

👁 Individual differences in susceptibility to hypnosis

Since hypnosis is a state that seems to have much in common with many other everyday states, anyone who can concentrate and follow simple instructions can, in theory, be hypnotized. They must trust the hypnotist and the hypnotist must be sufficiently skilled in the use of the correct hypnotic techniques. In practice, however, some people can be hypnotized far more readily than others. In fact, research shows that about 10% of the population are highly sensitive to hypnosis, about 10% of the population are very resistant to hypnosis, and the remaining 80% are susceptible to a greater or lesser degree (Hilgard, 1982).

A person's susceptibility to hypnosis can be assessed using one of a number of tests. The most widely used is the Stanford Hypnotic Susceptibility Scale (SHSS) (Hilgard, 1965), a 12-point behavioural test that comprises three phases:

- A brief discussion with the hypnotist to calm any fears or misconceptions about hypnosis
- A brief hypnotic induction to allow the participant to enter a hypnotic state
- A series of test suggestions that the participant either passes or fails.

To pass an item, the participant must not only comply with the suggestion, but must also feel that the action is involuntary and effortless. The suggestions used in the test range from simple 'motor' commands, such as 'your arm will now rise by itself' or 'you are unable to open your eyes', to more complex 'cognitive' suggestions that require participants to suspend disbelief or distort normal thought processes. Suggestions are also either 'positive' or 'negative' in nature. Cognitive suggestions include items such as 'behave as if you are weightless' and 'you can no longer hear, you are deaf'.

Being able to measure **hypnotic susceptibility** reliably has allowed researchers to investigate whether there are specific characteristics that will predict who will be susceptible to hypnosis. Although more research is needed, a general picture of susceptibility has begun to emerge:

1 *Hypnotic susceptibility is a stable personality trait:* Longitudinal studies, such as that conducted by Piccione et al. (1989), which tested the hypnotic susceptibility of college students, have found high levels of test–retest reliability over periods as long as 25 years. Individual susceptibility scores were very similar even when measured 25 years apart, suggesting that susceptibility is a stable part of our personality.

2 *Hypnotic susceptibility may have a genetic basis:* A study that compared the susceptibility to hypnosis of monozygotic (MZ) and dizygotic (DZ) twins found that MZ twins were far more likely than DZ twins to have similar scores on the SHSS, that is, to show higher concordance rates (Morgan, 1973). Given that MZ twins are genetically identical, this is evidence that hypnotic susceptibility may have a genetic basis.

There is also evidence that susceptibility may be related to subtypes of a particular gene, the COMT gene. So far, this research has only been carried out using male participants and so this may not be true for women (Lichtenberg et al., 2000).

3 *Structural differences in the brain may be related to susceptibility:* Research, including the classic split brain studies of Sperry (Chapter 1), has shown that the corpus callosum plays a vital role in coordinating the activities of the two halves of the brain, the hemispheres. One study has identified a region of the corpus callosum, called the rostrum, that is enlarged in those who are highly susceptible to hypnotic suggestion (Horton et al., 2004). A speculation might be that susceptible individuals inherit a particular

modification to the corpus callosum that affects communication between the hemispheres. This relates to the next possibility.

4 *Functional differences in the way that the brain works may be related to susceptibility:* Neuroimaging studies show that, under hypnosis, there is less activity in the 'rational' left hemisphere of the brain and more activity in the 'artistic' right hemisphere of the brain. It may be that those people whose right hemisphere is naturally more active are most readily hypnotized (Nash et al., 2009). This may also have implications for reporting on hypnotic states. Remember that Sperry's split brain patients (Chapter 1) could not comment on activities of the right hemisphere as language is contained within the separated left hemisphere. If, in the hypnotic state, the balance between the hemispheres is shifted, reporting by the verbal left hemisphere on the increased activities of the right hemisphere may be disrupted. As our self-awareness is intimately tied up with language, this might explain the apparent loss of self-awareness in hypnotic trances.

5 *Correlation studies show that specific personality traits are related to susceptibility:* It was once thought that people who are weak-willed, more compliant and obedient, or less intelligent are most susceptible to hypnosis, In fact, it seems that the critical characteristics include the ability to sustain attention and filter out distractions (Crawford et al., 1993), being more open to experience, having a more vivid imagination and being more fantasy prone, and having a greater ability to become deeply absorbed in activities (Hilgard, 1979; Lynn and Rhue, 1986; Nadon et al., 1991). These characteristics seem to be linked to an increased susceptibility to hypnosis.

Thinking scientifically → **How suggestible are you?**

The only way to know whether you can be hypnotized is to undergo hypnosis, but there are two tests that hypnotists use to see whether it is likely a person would be susceptible.

The magnetic force test
Just close you eyes and hold your arms out straight in front of you, with the palms facing. Now, imagine there is a magnetic force pulling your hands together – really try to feel those magnets tugging your hands towards each other. Concentrate on this image for one minute, then open your eyes. Have your hands moved closer together? This happens for about 70% of people. This group is considered more suggestible, and so probably more hypnotizable.

The eye-roll test

It is possible to see whether you might be susceptible simply by looking in a mirror. If more of the white, or sclera, shows when you look up, it is likely that you will be susceptible to hypnosis.

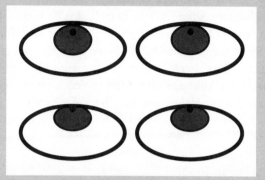

Figure 6.1 Eye-roll test

Of course, these are not scientific studies. Although findings from these tests seem to correlate with hypnotic susceptibility, correlations only show an association between two things, and not a cause-and-effect relationship. In particular, it is difficult to imagine a mechanism or process that links the whites of the eyes with hypnotic suggestibility.

The relaxed, focused, absorbed state associated with hypnosis has been used for centuries, with some success, to treat medical conditions, to reduce pain, to break undesirable habits and to unlock the unconscious mind during psychoanalytic psychotherapy. Charcot, a nineteenth-century neurologist, used hypnosis to treat psychological disorders, especially neurosis, and was a significant influence on his most famous pupil, Freud (who was then a medical student).

However, despite its long and successful application, academics, doctors and psychotherapists continue to argue over what hypnosis is, and what factors render people suggestible to the hypnotist's commands.

Since the 1960s, a vigorous debate, known as the state/non-state debate, has raged among theorists. On one side are the state theorists who all, in various ways, suggest that people's behaviour under hypnosis is a result of the hypnotic induction procedure inducing an altered state of consciousness (ASC). On the other side are the non-state theorists who are sceptical of this view. Instead, they suggest it is social influence that is responsible for people's behaviour under hypnosis.

State theories of hypnosis

Freud's view, along with others, was that hypnosis is a unique and altered state of consciousness, and this led him to use it in his psychoanalytic treatment of mental disorders, although it is notable that he eventually discarded hypnosis in favour of other techniques such as free association and dream analysis. Since then, a number of altered state theories (for example Hilgard, 1986; Bowers, 1992) have been put forward to explain the way that hypnosis works. Although they differ in detail, **state theories of hypnosis** centre around the view that hypnosis produces an altered state of consciousness that is qualitatively distinct from other states of consciousness.

Hilgard's neodissociation theory

Perhaps the most popular of the state theories is Ernest Hilgard's neodissociation theory (1986). In this, Hilgard suggests that hypnosis results in consciousness being split into two or more separate streams, each operating independently and divided by an 'amnesic barrier'. This theory was developed following a demonstration of hypnosis given by Hilgard to a group of students. During this demonstration, it became apparent that at the same time that one part of a volunteer's consciousness was hypnotized and unaware of what was going on, there was a second part of his consciousness that was not hypnotized. In contrast, this part was fully aware of what was going on in the hypnotized part of consciousness. It was as if a second stream of consciousness was watching the hypnotized stream, and so Hilgard (1978) termed this second stream of consciousness the **hidden observer**.

During the demonstration, a male student volunteer underwent a hypnotic induction. Once in a hypnotic trance, Hilgard gave the suggestion that on the count of three the volunteer would no longer be able to hear and would remain deaf until touched on the shoulder. After counting to three, Hilgard tested the volunteer's hypnotic deafness by making a series of very loud noises, including firing a starting pistol. Although the audience jumped, the volunteer did not react. A member of the audience then asked Hilgard whether, given that the volunteer was not really deaf, there was any part of him that knew what was happening. To find out, Hilgard said to the participant: 'Although you are hypnotically deaf, is some part of you hearing my voice? If there is, I should like the index finger of your right hand to rise as a sign that this is the case.' The finger rose. The volunteer immediately said: 'Please restore my hearing so you can tell me what you did. I felt my finger rise in a way that was not a spontaneous twitch.'

Intrigued, Hilgard placed his hand on the young man's shoulder to restore his hearing (the agreed sign) and told him that he would explain what had happened later, but first he asked the student to tell him everything he could remember. The young man reported that he heard Hilgard suggesting that he would be deaf on the count of three and that his hearing would be restored when a hand touched his shoulder. After this, he said, everything went very quiet and he could recall nothing until the time that his finger, seemingly spontaneously, lifted.

Hilgard then suggested to the volunteer, who was still hypnotized, that there was a hidden part of his mind that knew everything that had happened while he had been hypnotized, and that when his arm was touched, this hidden part would enable him to remember everything. Hilgard placed a hand on his arm and, sure enough, the student was able to report everything – the counting to three, the loud noises and the question from the audience about whether there was any part of him that could hear. He also remembered Hilgard asking him to raise his finger, so at last the volunteer understood why his finger had seemed to rise spontaneously.

Hilgard then lifted his hand away from the subject's arm to restore the hypnotic state and said: 'Please tell me what happened in the past few minutes.' The volunteer replied: 'You said some part of me would talk to you. Did I talk?' He was assured that he did and that everything would be explained to him once the session was over (Hilgard, 1978).

The cold pressor test and the hidden observer

This demonstration of the 'hidden observer' clearly suggested that consciousness could be divided, with one stream being hypnotized and unaware of what was happening while a second stream, which was not hypnotized, would be aware of everything that happened. However, it was limited in its usefulness. First, it was only a single case study and, as such, it was possible that the observed effects were unique to this volunteer. Second, this was only an observation, and conclusions about cause and effect cannot be drawn from observations. To test the theory, Hilgard needed to conduct an experiment.

Hilgard, Morgan and MacDonald (1975) used a pain tolerance experiment, known as the **cold pressor test**, to see whether hypnosis could reduce levels of reported pain. In this test, participants were required to immerse a hand in a tub of ice cold water for about a minute, a painful experience. They were asked to rate, every 10 seconds, how much pain they felt on a 10-point scale. Participants were divided into two groups; one group of participants were hypnotized and the suggestion was made that they would feel no pain, while in the control group, there was no hypnosis and no suggestion. The results showed that compared to the control group who reported maximum pain levels of 10 within 25 seconds, the hypnotized participants reported feeling far less pain, with mean ratings never exceeding two on the scale. The results from this study suggest that while this is a task that causes considerable pain, the use of hypnotic suggestion significantly reduced the experience of pain.

Hilgard used a variation of the cold pressor task to examine whether, at the same time that hypnotized participants reported low levels of pain, there was a second stream of consciousness, the hidden observer, that was aware of the real pain they were experiencing. In this study, the hypnotized participants were asked not only to report their conscious pain level verbally, but were also asked to use their free hand to press a key indicating whether any part of them was in pain. According to neodissociation theory, the hidden observer would use control of the free hand to indicate the 'true' level of pain. The results were striking. Although their verbal reports of pain were similar to the original results, the pain levels indicated by the 'hidden observer' reached an average rating of just over eight. These two very different reports of the same painful experience levels suggest that hypnosis can indeed induce a state of dissociation.

Other evidence of consciousness being divided

As well as experimental evidence of the type provided by Hilgard, there are other sources of support for the idea that consciousness can be divided in the way suggested by Hilgard and other state theorists. There are everyday examples, such as when you drive somewhere, only to realize afterwards that you cannot recall the route you took or whether or not you obeyed the traffic signals. One part of you drove and knew what was happening on the road, while another part of you daydreamed and was unaware. Alcohol and drugs can have similar consciousness-altering effects.

There are also more dramatic examples of dissociation, such as those that occur when hypnosis is used to regress clients back to an earlier age during psychotherapy. During age regression, one part of the hypnotized client's consciousness imagines returning to an earlier age, while another part remains in the present. However, perhaps the most dramatic example of the dissociation of consciousness occurs in a condition known as **dissociative identity disorder** (the original name for this condition was multiple personality disorder). In this condition, the patient's consciousness becomes pathologically dissociated into several streams as a way of coping with emotional problems. Each stream of the split consciousness takes on a different personality, with different voices, postures, and even dress. One personality usually dominates at a time, and is often unaware, or only dimly aware, of the existence of the other personalities. A well-documented example of this disorder is known as the 'three faces of Eve', which was reported by Thigpen and Clerkley (1957), and also made into a film of the same name.

Thinking scientifically → Defining altered states of consciousness

In Chapter 1 we reviewed some approaches to consciousness and awareness. The most straightforward model of consciousness distinguishes primary consciousness, similar to basic awareness and reactivity, from higher order consciousness, which possesses conscious self-awareness. In the classic hypnotized state, the person loses self-awareness, and the non-state approach would conclude that the effect of the social setting is to weaken this aspect of consciousness and allow the person to behave as if hypnotized. However, the state approach is more complicated. According to Hilgard's neodissociation theory, consciousness divides so that one stream retains awareness of what is going on. However, until interrogated by the hypnotist or researcher, the existence of the 'hidden observer' is unknown to the hypnotized person, that is, it does not represent self-awareness, and does not exert executive control during the hypnotic process. So it cannot be incorporated into simple models of consciousness, although it does have similarities with Sperry's ideas (based on his split brain studies; Chapter 1) of each hemisphere having a different type of consciousness. It may also be linked to dissociative identity disorder, when people develop multiple personalities, each of which is unaware of the other. However, each personality does seem to have its own higher order consciousness or 'self-awareness', something missing with the hidden observer.

We are a long way from explaining hypnosis or establishing the existence of any hidden observer. The jury is still out on whether hypnosis is an ASC, although it certainly poses problems for attempts to explain human consciousness. Also, given that psychologists have not yet managed to agree on a precise definition of consciousness, it is not surprising that there is little agreement on what constitutes an ASC. A particular problem with hypnosis is not being able to operationalize the concepts precisely, that is, to describe the procedures used to measure or assess the altered state. This poses problems when it comes to researching and evaluating theories of hypnosis; if the researchers are using different definitions and measures of altered states, then it is impossible to compare results.

◉ Non-state theories of hypnosis

We have seen that there is some evidence to support the traditional, altered state view of hypnosis. However, there are scientists, particularly social psychologists, who remain sceptical (for example Barber, 1969; Wagstaff, 1981; Spanos, 1986; Lynn et al., 1990). In their view, it is social pressures and the influence of the hypnotist that induce people to act in line with hypnotic suggestions, not an ASC. People may act 'as if' they are in an ASC because they believe that is how someone under hypnosis should behave and not because they are actually in an ASC. Remember the Orne and Evans (1965) study that demonstrated how participants only pretending to be hypnotized still followed the hypnotist's instructions? **Non-state theories of hypnosis** try to explain hypnotic phenomena using established psychological principles, as described below.

Social influence

What exactly are the social influences that non-state theorists believe are powerful enough to induce people to behave in line with the hypnotist's suggestions? There are two particular forms of social influence that could be involved, and with which you may already be familiar; conformity and obedience to authority.

Conformity and role playing

In life, we all play a variety of roles – son or daughter, sibling, head of school, soccer fan, teacher, boss, to name but a few. Each of these roles is accompanied by a set of norms (ways of behaving) that people conform to when they find themselves in that role. Non-state theorists argue that 'hypnotized volunteer' is a role like any other and, as such, is accompanied by a set of norms that lead people to feel and behave in a certain way.

There are two types of conformity, which, in different ways, may induce role playing in hypnotic procedures:

1 Normative social influence results in a type of conformity known as *compliance*. This can lead people to behave in the way expected of a 'hypnotized volunteer'. They do not really believe they are hypnotized, but wish to avoid the potential embarrassment of behaving in the 'wrong way' and so act as they think a hypnotized participant might.

2 Informational social influence produces a type of conformity known as *internalization*. This may be involved as people are often uncertain how to behave under hypnosis. When this is the case, they look for information to guide them. As most people's understanding of hypnosis is based on the state view, they believe that hypnosis will induce a trance-like state. In this state, they expect to behave in extraordinary ways in response to suggestions made by the hypnotist, and so they behave accordingly.

As Asch (1952) identified in his classic studies of conformity, the pressure to conform to a role is increased when we are being watched. The same is true under hypnosis – the pressure to conform to the role of 'hypnotized volunteer' is increased when under the scrutiny of others, which is why the presence of an audience at stage shows can produce such dramatic behaviours from volunteers.

It is important to understand that although these non-state theorists use terms such as 'role playing' to describe the behaviour of participants, they are not suggesting that people are faking a hypnotic response. They accept that hypnotized participants have unusual experiences, but they believe that it is social influence rather than an ASC that is responsible for these experiences (Spanos and Katsanis,1989).

Thinking scientifically → **Role playing and demand characteristics**

Pressures to conform to the role of 'hypnotized participant' are somewhat like the effect of demand characteristics found in other types of research, where the desire to be helpful leads participants to look for cues as to how they should behave. In hypnosis, the participant is also striving to be a 'good participant' and tries to behave in a way that will ensure the hypnosis is successful. This can be a problem for researchers. If a participant's beliefs and expectations about the way they should behave influence their behaviour, this could result in errors in the data, and false conclusions being drawn.

One method that researchers often use to minimize the effect of demand characteristics is deception. While this is generally an effective solution, providing the ethical issues attached to deception are addressed, in hypnosis research the use of deception is almost impossible. The true nature of the research is usually obvious as the hypnotic procedure cannot be disguised.

Another method that is used to control experimenter effects is the use of double-blind trials, in which the data is collected by someone other than the researcher, so eliminating the possibility of researcher bias. But this too is a problem in hypnosis research, as the person conducting the research delivers the suggestions and so cannot be blind to the purposes of the study.

Obedience to authority

The second source of social influence that could play a role in determining a participant's response to suggestion is known as 'obedience to authority'. You may have already read about Milgram's (1963) legendary research investigating people's responses to commands issued by those they perceive to be legitimate authority figures, if not, take a moment to read about the dramatic effects that perceived authority figures can have on people's willingness to undertake extreme behaviour. Although some people are reluctant to follow unreasonable commands given by authority figures, many do, even to the extent that they are willing to follow commands that would (apparently) kill others. Milgram also noted that the willingness of participants to follow instructions is increased when the authority figure is in close proximity. One explanation that has been offered for this behaviour is that people feel that the responsibility for the actions lies with the authority figure rather than with themselves – something Milgram termed an 'agentic shift'.

In many ways, this situation can be likened to hypnosis. Experienced hypnotists, who generally have great charisma, may be seen as legitimate and credible authority figures, and they work in close proximity with participants. So, it is possible that people's willingness to follow suggestions is merely the result of obedience, rather than an ASC. This obedience could either be explained by an agentic shift reducing the person's inhibitions, or it could simply be due to the fear of embarrassment or punishment that might follow if they were to disobey the authority figure, the hypnotist.

◉ State or non-state theories: which view is correct?

As we have seen, state theorists suggest that hypnosis produces an ASC, and it is this that is responsible for the behaviour we see. Non-state theorists propose that the behaviour under hypnosis is the result of social influence – conformity, role playing and obedience – rather than an ASC. As such, the effects of suggestion can be experienced without the need for a hypnotic induction procedure designed to alter the state of consciousness. But which view is correct? To resolve the debate, there are a number of lines of evidence we can draw on, from both behavioural studies and physiological studies that examine changes in the brain.

Behavioural evidence

Behavioural studies that compare the responses to suggestions of those who are high in hypnotic susceptibility with those low in hypnotic susceptibility have been the mainstay of scientific research in this area.

Real–simulator studies

Real–simulator studies developed to compare the behaviour of participants known to be high in hypnotic susceptibility (the 'reals') with that of participants low in hypnotic susceptibility, but who are told to act 'as if they were hypnotized' (the 'simulators'). The behaviour of all participants is assessed by an examiner who is blind to whether the participant is a 'real' or a 'simulator'. To ensure participants who are simulators are motivated in their efforts to play the role, they are told that if the examiner assessing their performance suspects they are only simulating hypnosis, the experiment will be terminated.

If, as the state theorists suggest, response to suggestion is related to an altered state of consciousness (ASC), research should reveal a difference between the two groups, as only the highly susceptible group will have been inducted into an ASC. If, as the non-state theorists argue, social influence can account for responses to suggestions, no differences should be found between the behaviour of those who are high in hypnotic suscep-tibility and hypnotized, and those who are low in hypnotic susceptibility but who are highly motivated to play the role of hypnotized volunteer.

Task performance

Many studies, across a wide range of tasks, have found no significant differences in the performance of those who are highly susceptible and hypnotized and those low in susceptibility but motivated to act as if they were hypnotized. This has been shown, for instance, in tasks such as eating onions while pretending they were apples, or following instruc-tions to throw what participants were told was 'acid' into the face of a research assistant. It has even been shown that highly motivated partici-pants could mimic the reduced pain levels of hypnotized participants in the cold pressor test (Spanos and Katsanis, 1989).

But while these findings seem to offer support for the non-state view, there have also been some studies that have found differences in behav-iour of reals and simulators. Perugini et al. (1998) looked to see whether behaviour differed dependent on whether an independent observer was present or absent. Both groups were given suggestions as to how they should behave via a tape recorder. The tape was played twice, once in front of an independent examiner and then again when the participants were alone. The results were clear. In front of the examiner, both the hypnotized participants and simulators complied equally with the suggested behaviour. But in the alone condition, a hidden camera revealed that while the highly responsive hypnosis participants continued to comply with suggestions such as petting imaginary cats or nodding their heads to imaginary music, the simulators did not. This would suggest that the simulators were responding to the social pressures of the situation, and of course these were only present when they were being observed. The presence of the observer made no difference to the reals, suggesting that they were not responding to the social aspects of the situ-ation but were perhaps in a genuine ASC.

Orne et al. (1968) also found a difference in the behaviour of reals and simulators. The suggestion was made that participants should touch their forehead whenever they heard the word 'experiment' mentioned during the two days that followed the session. Results showed that highly suggestible participants complied with the instruction far more often than the simulators.

Trance logic

We can also look at another type of research to see whether there are differences in the behaviour of reals and simulators. Trance logic refers to the ability of hypnotized participants to tolerate things that are logically inconsistent and would be challenged by people in a normal, waking state. Studies have shown that reals are able to hallucinate the presence of people who are not actually there, and even to hallucinate an image of a person sitting next to them when the person is actually standing on the other side of the room. When simulators are asked to do the same thing, they are far less successful.

Availability of information

This area of research looks at the availability of information about what occurs during hypnosis. If, as the state theories suggest, hypnosis is an ASC, people in an altered state would not recall what happened under hypnosis unless the suggestion is made that they will remember, but only when a specific cue is given. This might be the hypnotist touching the participant's arm, or saying a specific word at a later point. You may recall that failure to recall events occurring during hypnosis is called post-hypnotic amnesia.

Research shows that posthypnotic amnesia is generally found. However, a study conducted by Coe and Yashinski (1985) found that, without a suggestion being made under hypnosis that the person would later remember, posthypnotic recall could be improved if participants were simply told that a lie detector test would reveal whether or not they were lying. This suggests that the information is actually available to the participant and therefore it challenges the state view that hypnosis involves an ASC. Participants seemed to be behaving 'as if' they were hypnotized, rather than being in a truly altered state.

Physiological evidence

One of the problems with behavioural studies is that controlling all variables in the situation is difficult, and they are also open to the effects of demand characteristics. As we have seen, these are particularly important in relation to hypnosis. Physiological measures, in contrast, not only allow us to examine whether hypnosis differs from other states of consciousness, but also offer a more objective way of determining whether the effects of hypnotic suggestion are the result of an altered state of consciousness. By using appropriate technology we can look at the way the brain responds under hypnosis.

Suggestions are experienced as real

Functional imaging techniques, such as functional magnetic resonance imaging (fMRI) and positron emission tomography (PET), allow us to examine the changing levels of activity in different parts of the brain while a person performs a task. Studies using these techniques suggest that hypnotized participants genuinely feel the effects of suggestions as real (Crawford et al., 1993; Kosslyn et al., 2000; Raiji et al., 2005). For instance, when it is suggested that they will see colours, imaging studies show that the colour-processing part of the brain is active – despite there being an absence of any real colour. When they are told to imagine coloured objects in black and white, the colour-processing areas are less active. When it is suggested that they will feel pain, the areas of the brain responsible for detecting pain are activated, and so on. The evidence from these studies suggests that although there may be instances in which participants do respond in ways designed to please the hypnotist, in general participants are not just role playing. Brain changes match the instructions they are given.

Hypnosis induces a unique states of consciousness

The use of the electroencephalograph (EEG) in the study of brain activation and states of awareness was outlined in Chapter 1. This technique has also been applied to the hypnotic state, and provides evidence that while hypnosis produces brain electrical activity that is similar to conscious but relaxed states, there are distinct differences. Although hypnosis may appear similar to the drowsy state that precedes sleep, the alpha wave activity – which typically accompanies the drowsy, pre-sleep state – is greatly increased during hypnosis, particularly among those participants who are high in hypnotic responsiveness (Graffin and Lundy, 1995). The relationship between hypnosis and meditation has also been examined, as the two appear to share many of the same characteristics. Again, EEG studies show that the patterns of brain activity differ significantly in participants undergoing hypnosis and in those practising Buddhist meditation, both in terms of the brain wave activity and the brain regions involved (Halsband et al., 2009). This is further evidence for hypnosis as a distinct brain state, and possibly a distinct state of consciousness.

Hypnosis increases activation in the area responsible for executive control

If state theories, such as the neodissociation model, are correct and consciousness can be divided into different streams, there must be a region in the brain that is responsible for coordinating the various parts of consciousness – if there wasn't, we would not experience the world in a unified way. This is generally referred to as 'executive control', and many studies have identified that the area of the brain responsible for executive control is the prefrontal cortex. As its name implies, this is an area of cortex at the front of the brain, and is the area most increased in size in humans and other primates relative to lower animals. It is thought that this increase in the size of the prefrontal cortex is responsible for the higher cognitive abilities of primates.

If hypnosis results in the splitting of consciousness, we would expect to find an effect in the prefrontal cortex, and indeed Halligan et al. (2000) have found that during the induction phase, in which the brain is prepared for the suggestions that will be given later, the prefrontal cortex becomes more active, while the activity of other brain regions are suppressed.

Hypnotic suggestion reroutes signals in the brain in reals but not in simulators

Although it is clear that under hypnosis the executive area of the brain becomes more active in order to coordinate the divided consciousness, this does not explain the effects of suggestion. Recently, Oakley and Halligan (2009) hypothesized that hypnotic suggestion may work by inhibiting or disconnecting some brain processes from the executive control system.

To test this, Cojan et al. (2009) examined the brain activity of 18 participants, in a between-groups design involving three groups:

1 a hypnotized group to whom the suggestion was made that their left hand was 'paralysed'
2 an unhypnotized but pretending group, in which participants were instructed to pretend their left hand was paralysed
3 an unhypnotized, control condition in which no instructions were given.

The task itself was simple; each trial began by showing a cue on a screen which indicated whether the participant should prepare to press a button with either their left or their right hand. This cue was then followed by another image. If the image was of a green hand, the participants were told they should press the button, but if the hand was red, they should not press the button.

The group of most interest was the hypnotized group. Instructions to use their right hand produced activity in the brain that was similar to that of the unhypnotized group. However, when asked to use their left, hypnotically paralysed hand, the results were quite different. When the cue appeared that indicated they should *prepare* their left hand to press the button, the motor cortex fired up in the normal way, but when the instruction came to *actually* press the button, the motor cortex failed to send a signal to the area of the brain responsible for moving the left hand. Instead, the signal was redirected to an area of the brain known as the 'precuneus'. This is an area involved in, among other things, visualizing movement. So, the area of motor cortex that prepared the hand to carry out the movement connected to the area in the brain involved in visualizing the movement of the left hand, rather than the area involved in carrying out the movement of the left hand.

If we compare this to participants who were asked to fake paralysis, we find no such disconnection between these two regions. These results support the idea that hypnosis does have significant effects on patterns of brain activity. Figure 6.2 shows how hypnotized people who are told that their left hand is paralysed show brain patterns that differ from those who aren't hypnotized and from those who aren't hypnotized but are told to pretend their left hand is paralysed.

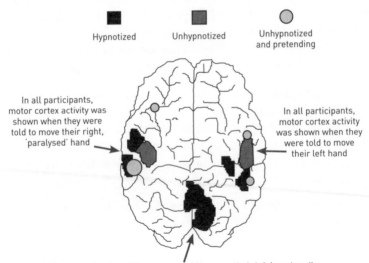

Figure 6.2 Your brain on hypnosis
Source: Adapted from Cojan et al., 2009

Hypnotic states and Stroop interference

We noted earlier that one of the characteristics of the hypnotic state is that attention is fully focused, and a number of theories have suggested that it may be differences in people's ability to control attention that underlie individual differences in hypnotic susceptibility (for example Gruzelier, 1998).

Some of the most interesting recent research has examined the effect of hypnotic suggestion on attentional control. An experimental paradigm that has been widely used for many decades to examine attentional control is the Stroop task (Stroop, 1935). In this, the names of colour words are printed either in the same (congruent) coloured ink ('red' ink for the word 'red', 'blue' ink for the word 'blue', and so on) or in a different (incongruent) ink colour ('blue' ink for the word 'red', 'red' ink for the word 'blue', and so on).

Participants are simply asked to name the colour of the ink the word is printed in. Although this may sound easy, to perform the task people need to attend to the relevant information (ink colour) and suppress or inhibit the irrelevant information (the meaning of the word), something most people find extraordinarily difficult. It seems that the meaning of the word is automatically activated and interferes with the naming of the ink colour. The difficulty participants have is reflected in the time it takes them to complete the task. In the congruent condition, they are much faster at naming the ink colours than in the incongruent condition, as in the incongruent condition, the automatic tendency to read the colour word interferes with the ability to name the colour of the ink.

The Stroop task provides clear evidence of the difficulties people have in controlling attention. But what would happen if, while under hypnosis, the suggestion is made that the participant is a native speaker of another language who could not read English, but who could still name the colour of the ink? If the state view is correct and hypnosis does alter brain function, then such participants would not be able to read the colour words and Stroop interference should be eliminated.

A study conducted by Raz et al. (2002) compared the performance of participants who were high in hypnotic susceptibility with those low in susceptibility. The key suggestion was that after hypnosis, they would see the words as gobbledegook, that is, they would not be able to read them, but would still be able to name the colour of the ink. The results showed that participants who were high in hypnotic susceptibility showed a similar speed of response in both congruent and incongruent conditions – in other words, they were behaving in line with the suggestion and the interference that is normally found when the meaning of the word conflicts with the colour disappeared. The same was not true of those low in hypnotic susceptibility, who showed the standard Stroop interference effect.

Studies such as this, which examine the impact of hypnotic suggestion on automatic processing, are important for two reasons. Not only do they show how hypnotic suggestion can be used to alter cognitive processes, but they also demonstrate a genuine effect that, because of the automatic nature of the process, would be virtually impossible for participants to fake. So, this evidence is clear support for state theories. Hypnotic suggestion appears to produce distinct and characteristic changes in patterns of brain activity.

Following this behavioural study, Raz et al. (2007) conducted the same study, but this time including brain scanning. Again, they found that participants high in hypnotic susceptibility were faster and made fewer errors in the incongruent Stroop trials than those who were low in hypnotic susceptibility. The imaging results also showed a marked difference between the two groups. When compared to the low susceptibility group, participants high in hypnotic susceptibility showed less activity in the occipital cortex, the area involved in processing visual information. During the incongruent trials, they also showed less activity in the area of the brain known as the anterior cingulate cortex. Again, this supports the state approach that hypnosis is associated with distinct changes in brain function.

Thinking scientifically → **Replication and reliability**

To date, compared with other areas in psychology, relatively little research has been conducted into hypnosis and suggestion. As such, many of the studies have yet to be replicated in order to establish reliability. In no area of science can a single study be taken as conclusive, however dramatic the findings. We can only be convinced if similar studies carried out by independent researchers find similar results.

When several similar studies have been done, a powerful technique can sometimes be used. This is a meta-analysis or meta-review. A meta-review uses statistics to combine the findings of different studies and produces an overall analysis using all the available data. The results of a meta-review are therefore more representative and reliable. Unfortunately, in hypnosis research, different techniques and methods are used in different studies and so it is not possible to do an overall meta-review.

What can we conclude?

At this point in the debate, it is simply not possible to conclude that either the state or the non-state view is correct. There is evidence to support both views. Behavioural and physiological differences between participants who are either high and or low in susceptibility, and between those who are hypnotized and those who are faking hypnosis, suggest state theorists are correct.

On the other hand, there is also evidence that some people succumb to hypnosis and comply with suggestions because they are responding to social influences, without any change in their state of consciousness. This would explain why people's expectations, motivations and rapport with the hypnotist play such an important role in hypnosis (Kirsch and Lynn, 1997). In short, it is likely that hypnosis involves, to some degree, both state and non-state processes, although proportions may vary with hypnotic susceptibility. It is for future research to determine the degree to which each is involved, rather than to determine which is right and which is wrong.

Thinking scientifically → **Ethics**

One of the greatest difficulties for researchers in this area is how to overcome the ethical challenges they face. We have already noted that deception is a problem. So too is obtaining full informed consent. Outlining the purpose of the study prior to the hypnotic procedure may influence the participant's behaviour. Also, hypnosis compromises a participant's right to withdraw at any time, and researchers should be concerned about the potential for psychological or physical harm that may follow hypnosis, particularly if extreme suggestions are made during the session.

There have been court cases in which people accused of bizarre or violent behaviour have blamed it on a previous experience of being hypnotized, usually in a stage show.

Applications of hypnosis

Whether we accept that people's responses to suggestion under hypnosis are due to an altered state of consciousness or simply the result of social influence, it is indisputable that hypnotism can provide a powerful tool for changing thought and behaviour in a wide range of settings. For generations, stage hypnotists have swung their pocket watches and made people behave in extraordinary ways, a practice now regulated by the Federation of Ethical Stage Hypnotists. But hypnosis is more than a stage act. Today, psychologists and healthcare professionals use hypnosis to change behaviour, block pain and recover memories. Hypnosis is also being used by researchers as a research tool.

Hypnosis and pain relief

Not everyone gains relief from pain under hypnosis, but there is considerable evidence that hypnosis can act as a form of psychological analgesia, particularly among those who score highly on the Stanford Hypnotic Susceptibility Scale. There is both anecdotal and research evidence showing that hypnosis helps during painful dental procedures, during childbirth, coping with the painful side effects of chemotherapy, and when experiencing chronic headaches, backaches and arthritis (Montgomery et al., 2001). There is even evidence that self-hypnosis can control pain during surgery (Olness, 1992).

The classic demonstration of the analgesic effect of hypnosis was provided by Hilgard et al. in 1975, in the cold pressor test. Participants were told they would feel no pain while their arm was immersed in a tank of ice cold water. Results showed participants who had been hypnotized were far more able to tolerate pain than those in the control group.

Hypnosis and recovered memories

Many hypnotists claim that the highly focused state of mind produced by hypnosis enhances the recovery of memories, and hypnotism has been used to tap into people's memories in two very different contexts – in the therapy room and during crime investigations:

- In *psychotherapy*, hypnosis is used to help recover memories that clients are often unaware they have. Psychoanalysts, in particular, use hypnosis to uncover repressed memories and childhood experiences. Hypnotic age regression is one of the more spectacular forms of memory retrieval. During age regression, a person imagines returning to an earlier age, while another part of the hypnotized participant's consciousness remains in the present. Hilgard (1978, p. 28) presented the following account:

I regressed a young women to childhood; she found herself lost in a department store where she had gone to shop with her mother and grandmother. She became frightened but accepted me as a sympathetic stranger when I comforted her. She saw her mother come to meet her and became happy … After she was roused from hypnosis, she said 'I felt sorry for that little girl, because I knew all the time that her mother was going to find her, but she did not know it.'

- In the *investigation of crime*, hypnosis is used to help recover the memories of victims or witnesses who know they have a memory of the event but simply cannot access it. This practice of using hypnosis to improve eye witness testimony and aid law enforcement is known as 'forensic hypnotism'. There are many reports of crimes being solved with the aid of hypnosis. For example, in 1976 the kidnapping of a busload of children was solved by hypnotizing the driver, who had not been taken captive. Under hypnosis, he was able to recall part of the number plate of the kidnapper's van. This was enough to enable the police to locate and rescue the children. The murder of a cellist at the Metropolitan Opera House in New York was also solved using hypnosis. One of the ballerinas saw a young man with the cellist prior to the murder. Under hypnosis, she was able to describe the man with sufficient accuracy to lead to his arrest.

But how accurate are these memories? It is important to remember that memories of past events are not like tape recordings (there are problems in judging the accuracy of eye witness testimony, and whether it can be influenced by leading questions and post-event information; recall under hypnosis is equally vulnerable to such factors). Memories are reconstructions that depend to some extent on imagination and inference. Just because a person can provide a detailed memory does not mean that memory is accurate. It is quite possible for the recovery of memories under hypnosis to result in **false memory syndrome**.

In the therapy clinic, experiences of age regression can feel very real but the memories that are recovered are generally difficult to verify objectively. A key problem is that there are usually no independent observers or witnesses. There is certainly some evidence to suggest that not all the memories that are recovered are accurate. For example, tests show that although childhood memories written down during regression appear to be written in a child-like scrawl, the writing the client produces often does not match samples of their actual handwriting that have been preserved from childhood.

This, of course, does not invalidate the memories, but does suggest that they may not be entirely accurate. Because of the potential problems in recovering accurate memories, both the American Medical Association and the British Psychological Society have concluded that memories recalled under hypnosis should be considered unreliable – they may be accurate, but should not be considered so unless they can be corroborated independently.

This has become a critical issue in relation to childhood abuse. Many psychological theories link adult psychological problems to physical or sexual abuse in childhood. Hypnotic age regression may uncover apparent evidence of such abuse. Such 'recovered' memories may allow the person concerned to resolve their psychological problems, but are also likely to lead to family breakdown and even criminal charges relating to abuse. It is therefore essential for recovered memories to be seen as accurate and reliable. However, as mentioned above, the consensus is that they should not be trusted unless verified by an independent source. A particular problem with hypnotic regression is that if the therapist believes that current psychological problems are linked to childhood abuse, then they are in a sense 'looking out' for it in the client's memories. They may consciously or unconsciously guide the person through their suggestions to identify instances of abuse that did not in fact happen – this is false memory syndrome. Unfortunately we often have no way of deciding conclusively whether recovered memories are true or false.

Likewise, in the courtroom, even when the witness provides great detail under hypnosis, this does not mean the memories are accurate, and apparent 'facts' must be treated with caution. It is quite possible that hypnosis has produced false memories, and it is not unknown for witnesses to provide memories that indicate the guilt of people who have subsequently been shown to have cast-iron alibis. Because of this, in contrast to the USA where courts accept evidence recovered under hypnosis, UK courts will not accept such evidence, although hypnosis can be used to help the police in their investigations.

So how might memories become distorted during hypnosis? There are two potential sources of distortion; the hypnotist, who may give leading suggestions, or use suggestive wording or intonation when delivering the suggestion, and the person being hypnotized. Research has found that people who are most susceptible to hypnosis are generally very imaginative and fantasy-prone, and more able to hallucinate (Wilson and Barber, 1983), so it is quite possible that these personality traits could affect the accuracy of recovered memories.

Hypnotherapy

Hypnotherapy has been shown to be a powerful tool in the treatment of psychiatric and emotional disorders. During a hypnotherapy session, the hypnotherapist works with the client in order to deal with deep, entrenched personal problems, by unlocking and reprogramming the unconscious mind.

Hypnotherapy has also been used with great success to help break negative patterns of behaviour, such as smoking or overeating. Some hypnotherapists do this by connecting a negative response with the bad habit, for example by suggesting under hypnosis that smoking will cause nausea. Others may focus on building willpower, suggesting to your subconscious you don't need or want cigarettes. Although directed, one-to-one sessions generally yield the best results in terms of long-term changes in thinking and behaviour, but hypnosis for the purpose of habit control can be conducted on a larger scale, perhaps during group seminars or by the use of self-help CDs. The success of these behavioural change programmes, however administered, has been shown to be related to levels of social support, and to the attitude and motivation to comply of the participant (Green and Lynn, 1995).

Hypnosis as a research tool

Recently, hypnosis has stepped away from the stage and the clinic and is now being used as a research tool to simulate psychological conditions (Schulz-Stübner et al., 2004). These include hallucinations, compulsions and delusions (Szechtman et al., 1998; Kosslyn et al., 2000), phantom limb syndrome (Willoch et al., 2000), amnesia (Mendelsohn et al., 2008) and pain (Rainville et al., 1997; Derbyshire et al., 2004). Creating 'virtual conditions' in a safe laboratory environment allows researchers to gain a better understanding of these states while avoiding some major ethical issues involved in studying such conditions in the real world. This, in turn, may lead to more effective diagnosis and treatment for a range of psychiatric and neurological disorders (Oakley, 2006).

Summary

- The hypnotic process consists of an induction phase, using fixed gaze, relaxation and imagery, or rapid induction, and a suggestion phase.

- The hypnotized phase is characterized by fully focused attention, extreme suggestibility, relaxation and performance of atypical behaviour.
- Susceptibility to hypnosis can be measured on the Stanford Hypnotic Susceptibility Scale. Susceptibility appears to be a stable personality trait with some genetic basis. There is some evidence for subtle differences in brain structure and/or organization in the highly susceptible. They also tend to be fantasy-prone, to have vivid imaginations, and to be able to sustain attention and filter out distractions.
- State theories, such as Hilgard's neodissociation theory, claim that the hypnotic state represents a qualitatively different state of awareness or consciousness. Non-state theories try to explain hypnotic phenomena using established psychological principles, especially those associated with social influence such as conformity and obedience.
- Hilgard's neodissociation theory hypothesizes that consciousness can be divided into two streams. One represents the hypnotized person, while the other, known as the 'hidden observer', is not hypnotized and remains aware of what is happening.
- Non-state theories use conformity, role playing and obedience to authority to explain hypnotic phenomena. Demand characteristics, beliefs and expectations are also important.
- Behavioural and physiological studies provide evidence for both approaches. The most convincing evidence for non-state theories comes from behavioural studies using 'reals' and 'simulators', showing that by using non-hypnotized participants, researchers can replicate many so-called 'hypnotic phenomena'. However, brain scanning and EEG studies have shown distinctive changes in brain function and organization associated with hypnosis. Areas involved include those involved with executive functions, while there is also evidence for a shift in arousal to the right hemisphere.
- It is probable that hypnosis involves a complex interaction between state and non-state processes.
- Applications of hypnosis include pain relief (analgesia), recovering memories either in a clinical setting or in relation to eye witness testimony, or as a clinical tool for treating addictions such as smoking. Hypnosis can be very effective in these areas, although there are serious questions over the reliability of memories recovered under hypnosis.

Glossary

Activation-synthesis theory of dreams: put forward by Hobson and McCarley, this theory proposes that dreams are a byproduct of the complex pattern of brain activity during REM sleep. Sensory and motor areas are active during REM sleep, and this accounts for the subjective imagery of dreams. Dreams are not acted out, as pathways from the brain to the body musculature are blocked during REM sleep. Dreams are often organized as the brain has an innate tendency to structure material in a systematic way.

Alpha waves: EEG wave pattern with a frequency of 8–12 hz characteristic of relaxed wakefulness.

Ascending reticular activating system (ARAS): structure running through the brainstem made up of millions of neurons and a key structure in modulating the arousal state of the brain. Centres within the ARAS are involved in the control of sleeping and waking.

Automatic processing: overlearned skills such as word processing or riding a bike. Automatic processing is rapid and occurs without conscious self-awareness.

Basal metabolic rate (BMR): a measure of energy consumption by the body. Small animals have a high BMR, and so conserve more energy through sleep. In general, BMR is positively correlated with total sleep time.

Behavioural approach: associated with Skinner, the approach focuses only on observable behaviour, and ignores internal cognitive and emotional processes in the brain.

Blindsight: phenomenon whereby patients apparently blind in one half of the visual field after damage to the visual cortex can still 'guess' at the location and movement of stimuli with above-average accuracy. Used as evidence for cognitive processing outside conscious self-awareness.

Body clock: *see* Endogenous pacemaker.

Cataplexy: sudden loss of muscle control while awake leading to physical collapse. A key symptom of narcolepsy.

Central sleep apnoea: *see* Sleep apnoea.

Chronotype: some people have biological rhythms that predispose them to be active and alert either in the early morning (morning types or 'larks'), or in the evening (evening types, or 'owls'). This is defined as their chronotype. Most people fall in between these extremes.

Circadian rhythm: a biological rhythm that has one cycle (one peak and one trough) every 24 hours. An example would be the sleep–waking cycle in humans.

Circannual rhythm: an infradian biological rhythm that takes one year for a complete cycle. An example would be hibernation in some animals, or possible seasonal affective disorder in humans.

Cold pressor test: used in studies of hypnosis and reported pain, this test involves immersing the hand in a bucket of ice cold water.

Commissurotomy: a neurosurgical procedure that cuts the corpus callosum, the major pathway connecting the two hemispheres of the brain. Used as a treatment of last resort for severe epilepsy, it also allowed Sperry to investigate the functions of the two hemispheres using these split brain patients.

Controlled processing: cognitive processes that require conscious self-awareness, such as planning and writing psychology books. Controlled processing is slower than automatic processing, takes more effort, and has limited capacity.

Core sleep: term introduced by Horne to describe a combination of REM sleep and deep NREM sleep. Recovery after sleep deprivation mainly involves these two components and so Horne considers them the most important sleep stages.

Corpus callosum: main pathway connecting the two hemispheres of the brain. It is cut as a last resort treatment for chronic epilepsy. *See also* Split brain patients.

Correlations: experimental approach that looks for associations between variables, for example seasonal affective disorder and day length. A significant correlation indicates a relationship, but cannot identify cause and effect; correlations may be influenced by uncontrolled variables.

Cortisol: hormone released from the adrenal cortex during states of stress. Helps cope with stress in the short term, but in the long term, high levels of cortisol can be damaging.

Delta waves: EEG wave pattern with a frequency of 1–3 hz, characteristic of the deep slow wave stages of NREM sleep.

Desynchronized EEG: an EEG brain pattern with no recognizable repeated waveform. A fast desynchronized pattern is characteristic of the alert waking state.

Diathesis-stress model: explains various disorders through an interaction between inherited vulnerabilities and environmental triggers.

Dissociative identity disorder: formerly known as multiple personality disorder, this psychopathology is characterized by the person taking on different personalities at different times. Each personality is unaware of the others, and the condition is seen as strong evidence for dissociated or separate streams of consciousness.

Diurnal: describes animals that sleep at night-time and are awake and alert during daylight hours. *See* nocturnal.

Divided field technique: introduced by Sperry and used to reveal the separate processing abilities of the two hemispheres. It can also be used with intact (neurotypical) participants. Stimuli in the left visual field are transmitted to the right hemisphere, and those in the right visual field are transmitted to the left hemisphere.

Dream work: in Freud's theory of dreaming, the dream work is made up of processes such as displacement and condensation that convert repressed impulses and urges (the latent content) into the dream imagery reported by the dreamer (the manifest content).

Dyssomnias: category of sleep disorders characterized by problems with the amount, quality and timing of sleep. These often lead to daytime sleepiness. Examples include insomnia, narcolepsy and sleep apnoea.

Electroencephalograph (EEG): reflects brain electrical activity. Recorded from a network of electrodes on the surface of the skull; *see also* Desynchronized EEG and Synchronized EEG.

Encephalization quotient (EQ): a measure of how advanced an animal's brain is compared to related species. More advanced animals such as humans and dolphins have a high EQ, and also have more REM sleep.

Endogenous: inbuilt or naturally occurring.

Endogenous pacemaker: inbuilt or innate (genetic) centres in the brain that function as body clocks, regulating the rhythmic activity of the body's physiological and behavioural functions. An example would be the SCN-pineal gland system that regulates the sleep–waking cycle.

Evoked potential: electrical signal recorded from the brain linked to the presentation of (or elicited by) a specific stimulus.

Evolutionary/ecological approach: an approach that tries to explain sleep patterns across the animal kingdom in terms of general lifestyle factors such as body size, brain size, habitat, sleeping place and so on.

Exogenous zeitgeber: external stimuli such as light onset that fine-tune the body's biological rhythms; they work together with endogenous pacemakers to synchronize biological rhythms with the outside world.

False memory syndrome: hypnotic regression can be used to uncover early memories. These sometimes involve childhood abuse and can lead to family trauma and criminal proceedings. However, there is evidence that such memories can be unreliable.

Fatal familial insomnia (FFI): a serious sleep disorder with familial (inherited) transmission. Chronic and almost complete insomnia develops in middle age and death usually follows a few years later. Associated with damage to the thalamus in the brain.

Functional magnetic resonance imaging (fMRI): technique using a brain scanner to record activity in different brain regions while participants perform various cognitive tasks. It is based on oxygen uptake by active neurons.

Hibernation theory: Webb used the analogy of hibernation to propose that a main function of sleep was to conserve energy. This would explain the correlation between basal metabolic rate and total sleep time.

Hidden observer: part of Hilgard's neodissociation theory of hypnosis. During hypnosis, consciousness splits into two streams. One, the hypnotized stream, is unaware of what is happening, while a second stream, the 'hidden observer', remains aware of all that is happening and can be contacted by the hypnotist.

Higher order consciousness: self-awareness, the experience of being able to think about our own experiences and the basis of our sense of identity. Contrasted with primary consciousness.

Hypersomnia: sleep disorder characterized by excessive daytime sleepiness and prolonged periods of night-time sleep. Primary hypersomnia is a chronic condition lasting months or years. Recurrent hypersomnia involves episodes of hypersomnia interrupted by episodes of normal sleep patterns.

Hypnotic suggestibility: there are large variations in individual susceptibility to hypnotic suggestion. Suggestibility can be measured using the Stanford Hypnotic Suggestibility Scale, and appears to be a stable personality trait that may have a genetic basis.

Hypocretin: brain neurotransmitter implicated in the sleep disorder narcolepsy. Some cases of narcolepsy appear to involve a reduction in levels of hypocretin in the brain, or an insensitivity of hypocretin receptors.

Infradian rhythm: a biological rhythm where one cycle lasts longer than 24 hours. Examples would be the human female menstrual cycle and annual hibernation in some animals.

Insomnia: problems with falling asleep, maintaining sleep, and/or early waking, leading to sleep loss and daytime tiredness. Categories include primary and secondary insomnia.

Isomorphic: REM sleep and dreams were once seen as isomorphic, in that referring to one implied referring to the other. The growing awareness that dreams could occur in NREM sleep led to the current view that dreams and REM sleep are not isomorphic. REM sleep is a particular neurophysiological state that can be objectively measured, while dreams are subjective phenomena that cannot be objectively measured.

Latent content: in Freud's theory of dreaming, the latent content of the dream is the underlying impulses and urges that are converted by the dream work into the manifest content reported by the dreamer.

Locus coeruleus: nucleus (collection of neuronal cell bodies) in the ascending reticular activating system (ARAS). Important in the regulation of REM sleep through the release of the neurotransmitter noradrenaline.

Lucid dreaming: an unusual state of awareness in which the dreamer becomes aware during the dream that they are dreaming. They can control the storyline of dreams and even make small consciously controlled movements of eyes and fingers during a dream. Lucid dreaming may be linked to the activation of frontal cortical areas usually inhibited during REM sleep.

Manifest content: in Freud's theory of dreaming, the manifest content is the dream imagery as reported by the dreamer. This is contrasted with the latent content.

Masking: used in priming studies. The priming word is masked so that it is inaccessible to conscious awareness, but even so can speed up the recognition of a semantically related target word.

Melatonin: hormone released by the pineal gland in response to external light levels. Melatonin has many effects on the brain and the body's physiological systems, and has been implicated in a range of biological rhythms. It has been tested as a possible treatment for jet lag.

Metarepresentation: another word for subjective self-awareness; *see* Higher order consciousness.

Narcolepsy: a sleep disorder, a dyssomnia that involves excessive daytime sleepiness and several characteristic symptoms; cataplexy (loss of muscle control), hallucinations when falling asleep or on waking, and sleep paralysis. It appears to have a significant genetic component.

Nerve impulse: all information is coded in the brain as nerve impulses, also known as action potentials. These are brief pulses of electrical activity conducted along and between neurons in the nervous system.

Neurobiological theories of dreaming: these theories try to explain the phenomena of dreaming through the neurophysiology of REM sleep, including patterns of brain activity. This approach sees the imagery of dreams as simply byproducts of brain activity during REM sleep.

Neuron: basic unit of the brain and nervous system, the neuron is a cell specialized to conduct electrical impulses. The brain contains between 20 and 100 billion neurons.

Nocturnal: describes animals that are alert and active at night and sleep during daylight.

Non-rapid eye movement (NREM) sleep: one of the two distinct forms of sleep. The deeper stages of NREM sleep are characterized by the presence of large slow waves in the EEG.

Non-state theories of hypnosis: this approach to explaining hypnosis tries to explain hypnotic phenomena using established psychological principles such as social influence, obedience, demand characteristics and conformity.

Noradrenaline: brain neurotransmitter associated with states of arousal. In particular, it is released by neurons of the locus coeruleus and plays a major role in the regulation of REM sleep.

Obstructive sleep apnoea: *see* Sleep apnoea.

Optional sleep: term introduced by Horne to describe the lighter stages of NREM sleep. Evidence from sleep deprivation studies suggests that optional sleep is not vital for restoration of brain or body. This is compared with core sleep – REM and deep NREM sleep.

Paradoxical sleep: old term for REM sleep, refers to the combination of deep sleep associated with a fast desynchronized (aroused) EEG.

Parasomnias: sleep disorders involving abnormal behaviours during sleep that do not lead to daytime sleepiness. Examples include sleepwalking, sleep terrors and REM sleep behavioural disorder.

Persistent vegetative state (PVS): describes patients in a comatose state, able to breathe alone but with no behavioural responses and an apparent lack of conscious awareness. Recent studies indicate that patients in PVS may show some conscious processing.

Phase advance: refers to a situation where the body clock is behind local time, for instance when flying west–east. It seems that phase advance is more difficult for the body to adjust to, and so jet lag after west–east flights can be worse than when flying east–west.

Phase delay: refers to a situation where the internal body clock is ahead of local time, for instance when flying east–west. Phase delay seems to be easier to adjust to than phase advance.

Pheromones: chemicals found in sweat and urine that function as chemical signals to other animals, indicating, for instance, sexual receptivity. They may also have a role as zeitgebers, synchronizing biological rhythms such as the menstrual cycle.

Polysomnography: the scientific study of sleep. In the sleep laboratory, polysomnography involves the recording of a variety of physiological measures during a night's sleep. These include the EEG, eye movements, body temperature, respiration and heart rate.

Posthypnosis amnesia: people may experience amnesia for events that take place while they are hypnotized. However, they often regain those memories when the hypnotist gives a prearranged signal.

Posthypnotic suggestion: refers to the situation when suggestions made by the hypnotist during the hypnotic session require the participant to act in a certain way when they emerge from their trance.

Primary consciousness: basic awareness of stimuli around us, characteristic of animals. Contrasted with higher order consciousness.

Primary insomnia: insomnia (sleep loss leading to daytime sleepiness) with no obvious cause such as a medical or psychological condition.

Priming studies: used to investigate attention and perception. Presentation of a semantically linked word speeds up the identification of a second target word; *see also* Masking.

Psychodynamic approach: associated with the work of Freud, this approach to explaining behaviour emphasizes the role of dynamic processes in the unconscious. It also assumes that early childhood experiences are critical in forming adult behaviour and personality.

Qualia: linked to consciousness, the subjective experiences of a particular sensation, such as the smell of coffee. We only have access to our own qualia, we cannot 'know' how other people experience the same sensations. One of the key problems in the study of consciousness.

Raphe nuclei: collections of neuronal cell bodies in the brainstem reticular activating system that are important in the regulation of slow wave sleep. Raphe neurons release the neurotransmitter serotonin.

Rapid eye movement (REM) sleep: one of the two distinct forms of sleep, associated with an aroused desynchronized EEG, eye movements and paralysis of the body muscles. Most of our dreaming occurs in REM sleep.

Real–simulator studies: experimental technique used to study hypnosis. People high in hypnotic susceptibility ('reals') are compared in various hypnotic procedures with people low in hypnotic suggestibility but asked to act 'as if' they were hypnotized ('simulators').

REM rebound: after REM sleep deprivation, participants show an overall increase in the amount of REM sleep when allowed to sleep normally. This is used as evidence for the critical role of REM sleep in brain restoration.

REM sleep behavioural disorder (RSBD): a sleep disorder found mainly in later life in which sufferers appear to act out their dreams. This should be impossible as the body muscles are usually paralysed during REM sleep and dreaming. Explanations include a genetic problem with this mechanism, focusing on the magnocellular nucleus and the neurotransmitter acetylcholine.

Restless legs syndrome: insomnia caused by an urge to relieve aches and pains in the legs by moving or rubbing the legs.

Restoration approach: an approach that tries to explain sleep patterns in terms of restoring physiological processes such as hormone levels and brain neurotransmitters.

Retinohypothalamic tract: pathway from the retina of the eye to the suprachiasmatic nucleus (SCN) of the hypothalamus. Transmits information about the amount of light entering the eye to the SCN, a key endogenous pacemaker in the brain. Allows for the synchronization of biological rhythms with the zeitgeber light.

Reverse learning theory of dreams: this theory, put forward by Crick and Mitchison, proposes that dreams are a byproduct of information processing during REM sleep. During REM sleep, the brain is eliminating unwanted memories and parasitic connections, and dream imagery is simply our experience of this process. Dreams are seen therefore as essentially random and meaningless.

Seasonal affective disorder (SAD): form of depression that occurs during the late autumn and winter months in some people. An infradian biological rhythm, SAD has been linked to a disruption of the link between internal body clocks and external zeitgebers caused by the shorter day length in winter. Exposure to bright light can be an effective treatment in some sufferers.

Secondary insomnia: insomnia in which a clear cause can be identified. This can be a pre-existing medical condition such as heart disease or asthma, or a psychological condition such as anxiety or depression. Stimulants and alcohol may also lead to secondary insomnia.

Serotonin: brain neurotransmitter with many functions. In particular, it is released by neurons of the raphe nuclei and promotes the onset of slow wave sleep.

Sleep apnoea: a sleep disorder, a dyssomnia associated with breathing problems. The sufferer experiences repeated pauses in breathing that cause waking. There can be many episodes each night. Obstructive sleep apnoea is caused by physical problems with the respiratory tract, while central sleep apnoea is a problem with the high level control of respiration by the brain.

Sleep efficiency: a technical measure of sleep. It is the ratio of time spent asleep against the total time spent in bed. Problems in falling asleep and night-time waking both reduce sleep efficiency.

Sleep exposure index: a measure of the safety of an animal's sleeping location.

Slow wave sleep (SWS): refers to the deeper stages of NREM sleep, characterized by large slow waves (delta waves) in the EEG.

Social cognition: area of cognitive psychology focused on how we perceive and process stimuli associated with other people. Basic to our ability to understand and interact successfully with others.

Somnambulism: technical term for sleepwalking. Somnabulism is a parasomnia found most commonly in children between 5 and 12 years old. It involves familiar behaviours and occurs in the deeper stages of NREM sleep. There is evidence for a genetic component, and other research focuses on brain development and incomplete control of arousal mechanisms.

Split brain patients: patients whose chronic epilepsy has been treated by severing the corpus callosum, so dividing the two hemispheres of the brain. Sperry's studies of split brain patients revealed much about the separate processing styles of the two hemispheres.

State theories of hypnosis: this approach to explaining hypnosis sees it as a special and unique state of consciousness. An example would be Hilgard's neodissociation theory.

Suprachiasmatic nucleus (SCN): a small set of neurons in the hypothalamus that have an intrinsic (inbuilt) rhythmic activity. Through a range of connections with other brain structures such as the pineal gland, the SCN has a major role as an endogenous body clock, controlling biological rhythms.

Synchronized EEG: an EEG brain pattern dominated by a regular waveform produced by the synchronized activity of many billions of neurons. Characteristic of states of drowsiness and the different stages of NREM sleep.

Theta waves: EEG wave pattern with a frequency of 4–7 hz characteristic of the drowsy state.

Threat simulation theory of dreams: put forward by Revonsuo, this evolutionary theory proposes that dreams are a time when animals and humans act out or simulate real-life threats and dangers, and practise coping responses. Evidence from studies of the content of human dreams provides only weak support for this model.

Trophic position: refers to an animal's position on the food chain, for example if they are carnivores or herbivores. Carnivores tend to be predators and herbivores tend to be prey animals. Trophic position has been linked to sleep patterns.

Ultradian rhythms: a biological rhythm with more than one complete cycle in 24 hours. An example would be the oscillation between REM and NREM sleep during the night.

References

Aldrich, M.S. (1998) Diagnostic aspects of narcolepsy. *Neurology*, 50, S2–7.

Allison, T. and Cicchetti, D.V. (1976) Sleep in mammals: ecological and constitutional correlates. *Science*, 194, 732–4.

American Academy of Sleep Medicine (2005) *International Classification of Sleep Disorders (ICSD-2)*. Newton, MA: American Academy of Sleep Medicine.

Ancoli-Israel, S. and Roth, T (1999) Characteristics of insomnia in the United States: results of the 1991 National Sleep Foundation Survey, I. *Sleep*, 1(22), S347–53.

Ancoli-Israel, S., Ayalon, L. and Salzman, C. (2008) Sleep in the elderly: normal variations and common sleep disorders. *Harvard Review of Psychiatry*, 16(5), 279–86.

Ardito, R. (2000) Dreaming as an active construction of meaning. *Behavioural and Brain Sciences*, 23, 907–8.

Arendt, J., Aldhous, J. and English, V. (1987) Some effects of jet-lag and their alleviation by melatonin. *Ergonomics*, 30, 1379–93.

Asch, S.E. (1952) *Social Psychology*. Englewood Cliffs, NJ: Prentice Hall.

Aschoff, J. (1967) Comparative physiology: diurnal rhythms. *Annual Review of Physiology*, 25, 581–600.

Aserinsky, E. and Kleitman, N. (1953) Regularly occurring periods of eye motility and concomitant phenomena during sleep. *Science*, 118, 273–4.

Banyi, E.I. and Hilgard, E.R. (1976) A comparison of active-alert hypnotic induction with traditional relaxation induction. *Journal of Abnormal Psychology*, 85(2), 218–24.

Barber, T.X. (1969) *Hypnosis: A Scientific Approach*. New York: Van Nostrand.

Barnier, A.J. and McConkey, K.M. (1998) Postyhpnotic responding away from the hypnotic setting. *Psychological Science*, 9, 256–62.

Beaumont, M., Batejat, D., Pierard, C. et al. (2004) Caffeine or melatonin effects on sleep and sleepiness after rapid eastward transmeridian travel. *Journal of Applied Physiology*, 96, 50–8.

Berger, H. (1929) Uber das Elektrenkephalogramm des Menschen. *Archives fur Psychiatrie und Nervenkrankheiten*, 87, 527–70.

Blackmore, S. (2003) *Consciousness: An Introduction*. London: Hodder & Stoughton.

Bonnet, M.H., and Arand, D.L. (1995) 24-hour metabolic rate in insomniacs and matched normal sleepers. *Sleep*, 18(7), 581–8.

Borbely, A.A. (2001) From slow waves to sleep homeostasis: new perspectives. *Archives Italiennes de Biologie*, 139, 53–61.

Borreguero, D. Larrosa, O., de la Llave, Y. et al. (2004) Correlation between rating scales and sleep laboratory measurements in restless legs syndrome. *Sleep Medicine*, 5(6), 561–5.

Bowers, K.S. (1992) Imagination and dissociation in hypnotic responding. *International Journal of Clinical and Experimental Hypnosis*, 40, 253–75.

Bowers, K.S. and Woody, E.Z. (1996) Hypnotic amnesia and the paradox of intentional forgetting. *Journal of Abnormal Psychology*, 105(3), 381–90.

Bruce, V. and Young, A.W. (1986) Understanding face recognition. *British Journal of Psychology*, 77, 305–27.

Cartwright, R. (1984) Broken dreams: a study of the effects of divorce and separation on dream content. *Journal for the Study of Interpersonal Processes*, 47, 251–9.

Chalmers, D.J. (1995) Facing up to the problem of consciousness. *Journal of Consciousness Studies*, 3(1), 200–19.

Chalmers, D.J. (1996) *The Conscious Mind*. Oxford: Oxford University.

Chemelli, R.M., Willie, J.T., Sinton.C.M. et al. (1999) Narcolepsy in orexin knocked out mice: molecular genetics of sleep regulation. *Cell*, 98(4), 437–51.

Cho, K. (2001) Chronic jet lag produces temporal lobe atrophy and spatial cognitive deficits. *Nature Neuroscience*, 4, 567–8.

Cho, K., Ennaceur, J.C., Cole, C. and Kook Suh, C. (2000) Chronic jet lag produces cognitive deficits. *Journal of Neuroscience*, 20, 1–5.

Chung, G.S., Choi, B.H., Lee. J. et al. (2009) REM sleep estimation only using respiratory dynamics. *Physiological Measurement*, 30(12), 1327.

Coe, W.C. and Yashinski, E. (1985) Volitional experiences associated with breaching posthypnotic amnesia. *Journal of Personality and Social Psychology*, 48, 716–22.

Cojan, Y., Waber, L., Schwartz, S. et al. (2009) The brain under self-control: modulation of inhibitory and monitoring cortical networks during hypnotic paralysis. *Neuron*, 62, 862–75.

Colman, A.M. (2001) *A Dictionary of Psychology*. Oxford: Oxford University Press.

Coren, S. (1996) *Sleep Thieves*. New York: Free Press.

Crawford, H.J., Gur, R.C., Skolnick, B. et al. (1993) Effects of hypnosis on regional cerebral blood flow during ischemic pain with and without suggested hypnotic analgesia. *International Journal of Psychophysiology*, 15, 181–95.

Crick, F. and Mitchison, G. (1983) The function of dream sleep. *Nature*, 304, 111–14.

Crowley, C.S., Acebo, C. and Carskadon, M.A. (2007) Sleep, circadian rhythms, and delayed phase in adolescence. *Sleep Medicine*, 8(6), 602–12.

Culebras, A. and Moore, J.T. (1989) Magnetic resonance findings in REM sleep behavior disorder. *Neurology*, 39(11), 1519–23.

Czeisler, C.A., Moore-Ede, M.C. and Coleman, R.M. (1982) Rotating shift work schedules that disrupt sleep are improved by applying circadian principles. *Science*, 217, 460–63.

Dauvilliers, Y., Maret. S. and Tafti, M. (2005) Genetics of normal and pathological sleep in humans. *Sleep Medicine Reviews*, 9(2), 91–100.

Davis, S., Mirick, D.K. and Stevens, R.G. (2001) Nightshift work, light at night, and risk of breast cancer. *Journal of the National Cancer Institute*, 93, 1557–662.

Dement, W.C. (1976) *Some Must Watch While Some Must Sleep*. New York: Simon & Schuster.

Dement, W.C. and Kleitman, N. (1957) Cyclic variations in EEG during sleep and their relation to eye movements, body motility and dreaming. *Electroencephalography and Clinical Neurophysiology*, 9, 673–90.

Dement, W.C. and Vaughan, C. (1999) *The Promise of Sleep*. Basingstoke: Macmillan – now Palgrave Macmillan.

Dennett, D.C. (1991) *Consciousness Explained*. Boston, MA: Little, Brown.

Derbyshire, S.W., Whalley, M.G., Stenger, V.A. et al. (2004) Cerebral activation during hypnotically induced and imagined pain. *NeuroImage*, 27, 969–78.

Domhoff, G.W. (1996) *Finding Meaning in Dreams: A Quantitative Approach*. New York: Plenum.

Durmer, J.S. and Dinges, D.F. (2005) Neurocognitive consequences of sleep deprivation. *Seminars in Neurology*, 25(1), 117–29.

Edelman, G. (1992) *Bright Air, Brilliant Fire: On the Matter of the Mind*. New York: Basic Books.

Floyd, J.A., Janisse, J.J., Jenuwine, E.S. and Ager, J.W. (2007) Changes in Rem-sleep percentage over the adult lifespan. *Sleep*, 30(7), 829–36.

Freud, S. ([1900]1955) The interpretation of dreams, in *Standard Edition*, vols 4 and 5. London: Hogarth Press.

Friedman, S. and Fisher, C. (1967) On the presence of a rhythmic, diurnal, and instinctual drive cycle in man: a preliminary report. *Journal of the American Psychoanalytic Association*, 15, 317–43.

Gold, D.R. Rogacz, S.R., Bock, N. et al.(1992) Rotating shift work, sleep, and accidents relating to sleepiness in hospital nurses. *American Journal of Public Health*, 82, 1011–14.

Graffin, N.R. and Lundy, R. (1995) EEG concomitants of hypnosis and hypnotic susceptibility. *Journal of Personality and Social Psychology*, 50, 1004–12.

Green, J.P. and Lynn, S.J. (2000) Hypnotism and suggestion-based approaches to smoking cessation: an examination of the evidence. *International Journal of Clinical and Experimental Hypnosis*, 548(2), 195–224.

Gruzelier, J.H. (1998) A working model of the neurophysiology of hypnosis: a review of evidence. *Contemporary Hypnosis*, 15, 3–21.

Hafeez, Z.H. and Kalinowski, C.M. (2007) Somnambulism induced by quetiapine: two case reports and a review of the literature. *CNS Spectrums*, 12(12), 910–2.

Hall, C. and Van de Castle, R. (1966) *The Content Analysis of Dreams*. New York: Appleton-Century-Crofts.

Halligan, P.W., Athwal, B.S., Oakley, D.A. and Frakowiak, R.S. (2000) The functional anatomy of a hypnotic paralysis: implications for conversion hysteria. *The Lancet*, 355, 986–7.

Hallmayer, J., Faraco, J., Lin, L. et al. (2009) Narcolepsy is strongly associated with the TCR alpha locus. *Nature Genetics*, 41(6), 708–11.

Halsband, U., Mueller, S., Hinterberger, T. and Strickner, S. (2009) Plasticity changes in the brain in hypnosis and meditation. *Contemporary Hypnosis*, 26(4), 194–215.

Heath, A.C., Eaves, L.J., Kirk, K.M. and Martin, N.G. (1998) Effects of lifestyle, personality, symptoms of anxiety and depression, and general disposition on subjective sleep disturbance and sleep patter. *Twin Research*, 1, 176–88.

Hilgard, E.R. (1965) *Hypnotic Susceptibility*. New York: Harcourt, Brace & World.

Hilgard, E.R. (1978) States of consciousness in hypnosis: divisions or levels? In F.H. Frankel and H.S. Zaminsky (eds) *Hypnosis at its Bicentennial: Selected Papers*. New York: Plenum.

Hilgard, E.R. (1982) Hypnotic susceptibility and implications for measurement. *International Journal of Clinical and Experimental Hypnosis*, 30, 394–404.

Hilgard, E.R. (1986) *Divided Consciousness: Multiple Controls in Human Thought and Action*. New York: Wiley-Interscience

Hilgard, E.R., Morgan, A.H. and MacDonald, H. (1975) Pain and dissociation in the cold pressor test: a study of hypnotic analgesia with 'hidden reports' through automatic key-pressing and automatic talking. *Journal of Abnormal Psychology*, 84, 280–9.

Hilgard, J.R. (1979) *Personality and Hypnosis: A Study of Imaginative Involvement*. University of Chicago Press: Chicago.

Hobson, J.A. (2002) *Dreaming: An Introduction to the Science of Sleep*. New York: Oxford University Press.

Hobson, J.A. and McCarley, R.W. (1977) The brain as a dream state generator: an activation–synthesis hypothesis of the dream process. *American Journal of Psychiatry*, 134, 1335–48.

Horne, J.A. (1988) *Why We Sleep*. Oxford: Oxford University Press.

Horne, J.A. and Pettitt, A.N. (1985) High incentive effects on vigilance performance during 72 hours of total sleep deprivation. *Acta Psychologia*, 58, 123–39.

Horton, J.E., Crawford, H.J., Harrington, G. and Downs, J.H. (2004). Increased anterior corpus callosum size associated with hypnotizability and the ability to control pain. *Brain*, 127(8), 1741–7.

Hublin, C., Kaprio, J., Partinen, M. et al. (1997) Prevalence and genetics of sleepwalking: a population-based twin study. *Neurology*, 48, 177–81.

Humphrey, N. (1986) *The Inner Eye*. London: Faber & Faber.

Hunt, H. (1989) *The Multiplicity of Dreams: Memory, Imagination, and Consciousness*. New Haven, CT: Yale University Press.

Irwin, M., McClintick, J., Costlow, C. et al. (1996) Partial night sleep deprivation reduces natural killer and cellular immune responses in humans. *The FASEB Journal*, 10, 643–53.

James, W. (1890) *The Principles of Psychology*. New York: Holt & Co.

Jouvet, M. (1967) Neurophysiology and the states of sleep. *Physiological Reviews*, 47(2), 117–77.

Jouvet, M. (1969) Biogenic amines and the states of sleep. *Science*, 163, 32–40.

Kales, A., Caldwell, A.B., Preston, T.A. et al. (1976) Personality patterns in insomnia: theoretical implications. *Archives of General Psychiatry*, 33(9), 1128–34.

Karni, A., Tanne, D., Rubinstein, B.S. et al. (1994) Dependence on REM sleep of overnight improvement of a perceptual skill. *Science*, 265, 679–82.

Kiefer, N. and Brendel, D. (2006) Attentional modulation of unconscious 'automatic' processes: evidence from event-related potentials in a masking priming paradigm. *Journal of Cognitive Neuroscience*, 18, 184–98.

Kirsch, I. and Lynn, S.J. (1997) Hypnotic involuntariness and the automaticity of everyday life. *American Journal of Clinical Hypnosis*, 40, 329–48.

Kitzinger, C. and Kitzinger, J. (2010) 'Giving voice to the voiceless': high-tech speculation, or basic respect? *The Psychologist*, 23(6), 450–51.

Koh, K., Joiner, W.J., Wu, M.N. et al. (2008) Identification of SLEEPLESS, a sleep-promoting factor. *Science*, 321(5887), 372–6.

Kosslyn, S.M., Thompson, W.L., Constantini-Ferrando, M.F. et al. (2000) Hypnotic visual illusion alters colour processing in the brain. *American Journal of Psychiatry*, 157, 1279–84.

LaBerge, S. (1985) *Lucid Dreaming*. Los Angeles: Jeremy Tarcher.

Lavie, P. (1996) *The Enchanted World of Sleep*. New Haven, CT: Yale University Press.

Lavie, P., Malhotra, A. and Pillar, G. (2002) *Sleep Disorders: Diagnosis, Management and Treatment: A Handbook for Clinicians*. London: Martin Dunitz.

Lecendreux, M., Bassetti, C., Dauvilliers, Y. et al. (2003) HLA and genetic susceptibility to sleepwalking. *Molecular Psychiatry*, 8, 114–17.

Lehrman, R. and Weiss, E.J. (1943) Schizophrenia in cryptogenic narcolepsy. *Psychiatric Quarterly*, 17, 135–44.

Lesku, J.A., Roth II, T.C., Amlaner, C.J. and Lima, S.L. (2006) A phylogenetic analysis of sleep architecture in mammals: the integration of anatomy, physiology, and ecology. *American Naturalist*, 168(4), 441–53.

Lesku, J.A., Roth II, T.C., Rattenborg, N.C. et al. (2008) Phylogenetics and the correlates of mammalian sleep: a reappraisal. *Sleep Medicine Reviews*, 12, 229–44.

Libet, B., Gleason, C.A., Wright, E.W. and Pearl, D.K. (1983) Time of conscious intention to act in relation to onset of cerebral activity (readiness potential): the unconscious initiation of a freely voluntary act. *Brain*, 106, 623–42.

Lichtenberg, P., Bachner-Melman, R., Gritsenko, I. and Ebstein, R.P. (2000) Exploratory association study between catechol-O-methyltransferase (COMT) high/low enzyme activity polymorphism and hypnotizability. *American Journal of Medical Genetics*, 96(6), 771–4.

Lilly, J.C. (1964) Animals in aquatic environments: adaptations of mammals to the ocean. In D.B. Dill (ed.) *Handbook of Physiology: Environment*. Washington, DC: American Physiology Society.

Lin, L., Faraco, J., Li, R. et al. (1999) The sleep disorder canine narcolepsy is caused by a mutation in the hypocretin (orexin) receptor 2 gene. *Cell*, 98, 365–76.

Loomis, A.L., Harvey, E.N. and Hobart, G.A. (1937) Cerebral states during sleep as studied by human brain potentials. *Journal of Experimental Psychology*, 21(2), 127–44.

Lopez, H.H., Bracha, A.S. and Bracha, H.S. (2002) Evidence based complementary interventions for insomnia. *Hawaii Medical Journal*, 61(9), 192–213.

Lyamin, O.I., Manger, P.R., Ridgway, S.H. et al. (2008) Cetacean sleep: an unusual form of mammalian sleep. *Neuroscience and Biobehavioral Reviews*, 32, 1451–84.

Lynn, S.J. and Rhue, J.W. (1986) The fantasy-prone person: hypnosis, imagination, and creativity. *Journal of Personality and Social Psychology*, 51(2), 404–8.

Lynn, S.J., Rhue, J.W. and Weekes, J. (1990) An integrative model of hypnotic involuntariness. In R. van Dyck, P. Spinhoven, A.Van der Does et al. (eds) *Hypnosis: Current Theory, Research and Practice*. Amsterdam: VU University Press.

MacEwen, B.S. (2000) The neurobiology of stress: from serendipity to clinical relevance. *Brain Research*, 886(1/2), 172–89.

Malcolm-Smith, S. and Solms, M. (2004) Incidence of threat in dreams: a response to Revonsuo's threat simulation theory. *Dreaming*, 14(4), 220–9.

Meddis, R. (1975) On the function of sleep. *Animal Behaviour*, 23, 679–91.

Mendelsohn, A., Chalamish, Y., Solomonovich, A. and Dudai, Y. (2008) Mesmerizing memories: brain substrates of episodic memory suppression in post-hypnotic amnesia. *Neuron*, 57, 159–70.

Mersch, P.P., Middendorp, H.M., Bouhuys, A.L. et al. (1999) Seasonal affective disorder and latitude: a review of the literature. *Journal of Affective Disorders*, 53, 35–48.

Mignot, E. (1998) Genetic and familial aspects of narcolepsy. *Neurobiology*, 50, S16–22.

Mignot, E. (2001) A commentary on the neurobiology of the hypocretin/orexin system. *Neuropsychopharmacology*, 25(5), S5–13.

Mignot, E., Hayduk, R., Grumet, F.C. et al. (1997) HLA DQB1*0602 is associated with cataplexy in 509 narcoleptic patients. *Sleep*, 20(1), 1012–20.

Milgram, S. (1963) Behavioural study of obedience. *Journal of Abnormal and Social Psychology*, 67(4), 371–8.

Montgomery, G.H., Du-Hamel, K.N. and Redd W.H. (2001) A meta-analysis of hypnotically induced analgesia: How effective is hypnosis? *International Journal of Clinical and Experimental Hypnosis*, 48(2), 138–53.

Monti, M.M. and Owen, A.M. (2010) The aware mind in the motionless body. *The Psychologist*, 23(6), 478–81.

Morgan, A.H. (1973) The heritability of hypnotic susceptibility in twins. *Journal of Abnormal Psychology*, 82, 55–61.

Morgan, E. (1995) Measuring time with a biological clock. *Biological Sciences Review*, 7, 2–5.

Morin, C.M. and Mimeault, V. (1999) Self-help treatment for insomnia: bibliotherapy with and without professional guidance. *Journal of Consulting and Clinical Psychology*, 67(4), 511–19.

Moruzzi, G. and Magoun, H.W. (1949) Brain stem reticular formation and activation of the EEG. *Electroencephalography and Clinical Neurophysiology*, 1, 455–73.

Mukhametov, L.M., Supin, A.Y. and Polyakova, I.G. (1977) Interhemispheric asymmetry of the electroencephalographic sleep pattern in dolphins. *Brain Research*, 134, 581–4.

Nadon, R., Hoyt, I.P., Register, P.A. and Kihlstrom, J.F. (1991) Absorption and hypnotizability: context effects reexamined. *Journal of Personality and Social Psychology*, 60(1), 144–53.

Nash, M.R., Perez, N., Tasso, A. and Levy, J. (2009) Clinical research on the utility of hypnosis in the prevention, diagnosis, and treatment of medical and psychiatric disorders. *International Journal of Clinical and Experimental Hypnosis*, 57(4), 443–50.

Neilsen, T. and Germaine, A. (2000) Post-traumatic nightmares as a dysfunctional state. *Behavioural and Brain Sciences*, 23, 978–9.

Nishino, S., Ripley, B., Overeem, S. et al. (2000) Hypocretin (orexin) transmission in human narcolepsy. *The Lancet*, 355, 39–40.

Novelli, L., Ferri, R. and Bruni, O. (2009) Sleep classification according to AASM and Rechstaffen and Kales: effect on sleep scoring parameters of children and adolescents. *Journal of Sleep Research*, 19, 238–47.

Oakley, D.A. (2006) Hypnosis as a tool in research: experimental psychopathology. *Contemporary Hypnosis*, 23(1): 3–14.

Oakley, D.A. and Halligan, P.W. (2009) Hypnotic suggestion and cognitive neuroscience. *Trends in Cognitive Sciences*, 13(6), 264–70.

Ohayon, M.M., Carskadon, M.A., Guilleminault, C. and Vitiello, M.V. (2004) Meta-analysis of quantitative sleep parameters from childhood to old age in healthy individuals: developing normative sleep values across the human lifespan. *Sleep*, 27(7), 1255–73.

Oliviero, A. (2008) Why do some people sleepwalk? *Scientific American Mind*, February.

Olness, J.M. (1992) Hypnosis: the power of attention. In G. Goleman and J. Gurin (eds) *Mind/Body Medicine*. Yonkers, NY: Consumer Reports Books.

Orne, M.T. and Evans, F.J. (1965) Social control in the psychological experiment: antisocial behaviour and hypnosis. *Journal of Personality and Social Psychology*, 95, 189–200.

Orne, M.T., Sheehan, P.W. and Evans, F.J. (1968) The occurrence of posthypnotic behavior outside the experimental setting. *Journal of Personality and Social Psychology*, 26, 217–21.

Oswald, I. (1969) Human brain protein, drugs and dreams. *Nature*, 223, 893–7.

Oswald, I. (1980) *Sleep*, 4th edn. Harmondsworth: Penguin Books.

Owen, A.M. and Coleman, M.R. (2008) Functional neuroimaging of the vegetative state. *Nature Reviews of Neuroscience*, 9, 235–43.

Owen, A.M., Coleman, M.R., Boly, M. et al. (2006) Detecting awareness in the vegetative state. *Science*, 303, 1402.

Perugini, E.W., Kirsch, I., Allen, S.T. et al. (1998) Surreptitious observation of responses to hypnotically suggested hallucinations: a test of the compliance hypothesis. *International Journal of Clinical and Experimental Hypnosis*, 46(2), 191–203.

Phillips, B., Magan, L., Gerhardstein, C. and Cecil, B. (1991) Shift work, sleep quality and worker health: a study of police officers. *Southern Medical Journal*, 84(10), 1176–84.

Piccione, C., Hilgard, E.R. and Zimbardo, P.G. (1989) On the degree of stability and measured hypnotizability over a 25-year period. *Journal of Personality and Social Psychology*, 56, 289–95.

Raij, T.R., Numminen, J., Narvanen, S. et al. (2005) Brain correlates of subjective reality of physically and psychologically induced pain. *Proceedings of the National Academy of Sciences*, 102(6), 2147–51.

Rainville, P., Duncan, G.H., Price, D.D. et al. (1997) Pain affect encoded in the human anterior cingulate but not somatosensory cortex. *Science*, 277: 988–71.

Rattenborg, N.C., Martinez-Gonzalez, D. and Lesku, J.A. (2009) Avian sleep homeostasis: convergent evolution of complex brains, cognition and sleep functions in mammals and birds. *Neuroscience and Biobehavioral Reviews*, 33, 253–70.

Rattenborg, N.C., Voirin, B., Vyssotski, A.I. et al. (2008) Sleeping outside the box: electroencephalographic measures of sleeping sloths inhabiting a rainforest. *Biology Letters*, 4(4), 402–5.

Raz, A., Kirsch, L., Pollard, J. and Nitkin-Kaner, Y. (2007) Suggestion reduces the Stroop effect. *Psychological Science*, 17(2), 91–5.

Raz, A., Shapiro, T., Fan, J. and Posner, M.I. (2002) Hypnotic suggestion and the modulation of Stroop interference. *Archives of General Psychiatry*, 59, 1155–61.

Recht, L.D., Lew, R.A. and Schwartz, W.J. (1995) Baseball teams beaten by jet lag. *Nature*, 377–8.

Rechtschaffen, A. and Kales, A. (1968) *A Manual of Standardised Terminology, Techniques, and Scoring System for Sleep Stages of Human Subjects*. Washington, DC: Washington Public Health Service, US Government Printing Office.

Rechtschaffen, A., Gilliland, M.A., Bergmann, B.M. and Winter, J.B. (1983) Physiological correlates of prolonged sleep deprivation in rats. *Science*, 221, 182–4.

Rees, G. (2007) Neural correlates of the contents of visual awareness in humans. *Philosophical Transactions of the Royal Society B – Biological Sciences*, 362, 877–86.

Revonsuo, A. (2000) The reinterpretation of dreams: an evolutionary hypothesis of the function of dreaming. *Behavioural and Brain Sciences*, 23, 793–1121.

Rial, R.V., Nicolau, M.C., Akaarir, M. et al. (2007) The trivial function of sleep. *Sleep Medicine Reviews*, 11, 311–25.

Russell, M.J., Switz, G.M. and Thompson, K. (1980) Olfactory influences on the human menstrual cycle. *Pharmacology, Biochemistry and Behavior*, 13, 737–8.

Sack, R.L., Auckley, D., Auger, R.R. et al. (2007) Circadian rhythm sleep disorders: part I, basic principles, shift work and jet lag disorders: an American Academy of Sleep Medicine review, *Sleep*, 30(11), 1460–83.

Savage, V.M. and West, G.B. (2007) A quantitative theoretical framework for understanding mammalian sleep. *Proceedings of the National Academy of Sciences*, 104(3), 1051–6.

Schenck, C.H. and Mahowald, M.W. (1996) REM sleep parasomnias. *Neurologic Clinics*, 14(4), 697–720.

Schiffrin, R.M. and Schneider, W. (1977) Controlled and automatic human information processing: II. Perceptual learning, automatic attending and a general theory. *Psychological Review*, 84, 127–90.

Schulz-Stübner, S., Krings, T., Meister, I.G. et al. (2004) Clinical hypnosis modulates functional magnetic resonance imaging signal intensities and pain perception in a thermal stimulation paradigm. *Regional Anesthesia and Pain Medicine*, 29(6), 549–56.

Serafetinides, E.A., Shurley, J.T. and Brooks, R.E. (1972) Electroencephalogram of the pilot whale, *Globicephala scammoni*, in wakefulness and sleep: lateralization aspects. *International Journal of Psychobiology*, 2, 129–35.

Shapiro, C.M., Bortz, R., Mitchell, D. et al. (1981) Slow-wave sleep: a recovery period after exercise. *Science*, 214, 1253–4.

Siffre, M. (1975) Six months alone in a cave. *National Geographic*, 147, 426–35.

Society for Science and the Public (1954) Sleepwalking cause. *The Science Newsletter*, 27 February, 132.

Soehner, A.M., Kennedy, K.S. and Monk, T.H. (2007) Personality correlates with sleep-wake variables. *Chronobiology International*, 24(5), 889–903.

Soon, C.S., Brass, M., Heinze, H.-J. and Haynes, J.-D. (2008) Unconscious determinants of free decisions in the human brain. *Nature Neuroscience*, 11(5), 543–45.

Spanos, N.P. (1986) Hypnosis and the modification of hypnotic susceptibility: a social psychological perspective. In P. Naish (ed.) *What is Hypnosis?* Philadelphia: Open University Press.

Spanos, N.P. and Katsanis, J. (1989) Effects of instructional set on attributions of nonvolition during hypnotic and nonhypnotic analgesia. *Journal of Personality and Social Psychology*, 56(2), 182–8.

Sperry, R.W. (1964) The great cerebral commissure. *Scientific American*, 210, 42–8.

Sperry, R.W. and Gazzaniga, M.S. (1967) Language following surgical disconnection of the hemispheres. In C.H. Millikan and F.L. Darley (eds) *Brain Mechanisms Underlying Speech and Language*. New York: Grune & Stratton.

Stephan, K.K. and Zucker, I. (1972) Circadian rhythms in drinking behaviour and locomotor activity of rats are eliminated by hypothalamic lesions. *Proceedings of the National Academy of Sciences*, 60, 1583–6.

Strauch, I. and Meier, B. (1996) *In Search of Dreams: Results of Experimental Dream Research*. Albany: State University of New York Press.

Stroop, J.R. (1935) Studies of interference in serial verbal reactions. *Journal of Experimental Psychology*, 18, 643–62.

Szechtman, H., Woody, E., Bowers, K.S. and Nahmias, C. (1998) Where the imaginal appears real: a positron emission tomography study of auditory hallucinations. *Proceedings of the National Academy of Sciences*, 95, 1956–60.

Thigpen, C.H. and Clerkley, H. (1957) *The Three Faces of Eve*. New York: McGraw-Hill.

Van de Laar, M., Verbeek, I., Pevernaigie, D. et al. (2010) The role of personality traits in insomnia. *Sleep Medicine Review*, 14(1), 61–8.

Van Dongen, H.P., Vitellaro, K.M. and Dinges, D.F. (2005) Individual differences in adult human sleep and wakefulness: leitmotif for a research agenda. *Sleep*, 20(4), 480–96.

Verheijde, J.l., Rady, M.Y. and McGregor, J.L. (2009) Brain death, states of impaired consciousness, and physician-assisted death for end-of-life organ donation and transplantation. *Medicine, Health Care and Philosophy*, 12, 409–21.

Vitiello, M.V. (2006) Sleep in normal aging. *Sleep Medicine Clinics*, 1, 171–6.

Vogel, G. (1960) Studies in psychophysiology of dreams (II), the dream of narcolepsy. *Archives of General Psychiatry*, 3, 421–8.

Wagstaff, G.F. (1981) *Hypnotism: Compliance, Belief and Doubt*. New York: St Martins Press.

Walker, M.P. and Stickgold, R. (2004) Sleep-dependent learning and memory consolidation. *Neuron*, 121–33.

Walker, M.P., Brakefield, T., Morgan, A. et al. (2002) Practice with sleep makes perfect: sleep-dependent motor skill learning. *Neuron*, 35, 205–11.

Watson, N.F., Goldberg, J. Arguelles, L. and Buchwald, D. (2006). Genetic and environmental influences on insomnia, daytime sleepiness, and obesity in twins. *Sleep*, 29(5), 645–9.

Webb, W.B. (1982) Sleep and biological rhythms. In W.B. Webb (ed.) *Biological Rhythms, Sleep and Performance*. Chichester: Wiley.

Weiskrantz, L. (2002) Prime sight and blindsight. *Consciousness and Cognition*, 11, 568–81.

Weiskrantz, L., Warrington, E., Sanders, M. and Marshall, J. (1974) Visual capacity in the hemianoptic field following a restricted occipital ablation. *Brain*, 97, 709–28.

Wickens, A. (2009) *Introduction to Biopsychology*, 3rd edn. Harlow, Pearson Education.

Willoch, F., Rosen, G., Tolle, T.R. et al. (2000) Phantom limb in the human brain: unravelling neural circuitries of phantom limb sensations using positron emission tomography. *Annals of Neurology*, 48, 842–9.

Wilson, S.C. and Barber, T.X. (1983) The fantasy-prone personality: implications for understanding imagery, hypnosis, and parapsychological phenomena. In A.A. Sheikh (ed.) *Imagery: Current Theory, Research and Application*. New York: Wiley.

Wolfson, A.R. and Carskadon, M.A. (1998) Sleep schedules and daytime functioning in adolescents. *Child Development*, 69(4), 875–87.

Wu, M.N., Koh, K., Yue, Z. et al. (2008) A genetic screen for sleep and circadian mutants reveals mechanisms underlying regulation of sleep in Drosophila. *Sleep*, 31(4), 465–72.

Zadra, A. and Donderi, D. (2000) Threat perceptions and avoidance in recurrent dreams. *Behavioural and Brain Sciences*, 23, 1017–18.

Zager, A., Andersen, M.L., Ruiz, F.S. et al. (2007) Effects of acute and chronic sleep loss on immune modulation in rats. *Regulatory, Integrative and Comparative Physiology*, 293, R504–9.

Zepelin, H. and Rechtschaffen, A. (1974) Mammalian sleep, longevity and energy metabolism. *Brain and Behavioral Evolution*, 10, 425–70.

Index

Reading guide

This table identifies where in the book you'll find relevant information for those of you studying or teaching A-level. You should also, of course, refer to the Index and the Glossary, but navigating a book for a particular set of items can be awkward and we found this table a useful tool when editing the book and so include it here for your convenience.

Topic	Specification		Page
	AQA(A)	WJEC	
Apnoea	x		85–6
Circadian rhythm	x	x	28–9, 32–4
Disruption of rhythms – jet lag	x	x	39–41
Disruption of rhythms – shiftwork	x	x	34–9
Endogenous pacemaker	x	x	25–9, 32–4
Evolutionary/ecological approach	x	x	56–62
Exogenous zeitgeber	x	x	26–30, 35–8
Hypersomnia		x	90–3
Infradian rhythm	x	x	29–30
Life span changes and sleep	x		70–2
Narcolepsy	x	x	93–100
Non-state explanation of hypnosis		x	140–51
Personality	x		83–4
Primary insomnia	x	x	78–81
Restoration theory	x	x	62–9
Secondary insomnia	x	x	81–90
Sleepwalking	x		101–5
State explanation of hypnosis		x	136–40
Ultradian rhythm	x	x	30–2